Conditioning for Dancers

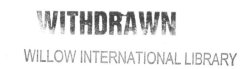

UNIVERSITY PRESS OF FLORIDA

Florida A&M University, Tallahassee
Florida Atlantic University, Boca Raton
Florida Gulf Coast University, Ft. Myers
Florida International University, Miami
Florida State University, Tallahassee
New College of Florida, Sarasota
University of Central Florida, Orlando
University of Florida, Gainesville
University of North Florida, Jacksonville
University of South Florida, Tampa
University of West Florida, Pensacola

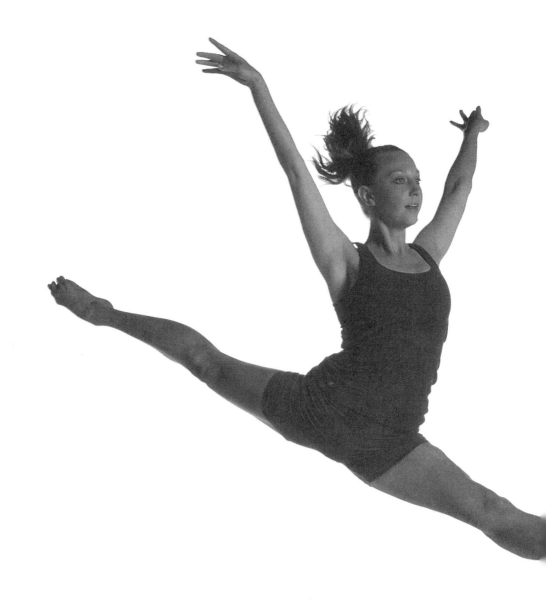

UNIVERSITY PRESS OF FLORIDA

Gainesville · Tallahassee · Tampa · Boca Raton · Pensacola · Orlando · Miami · Jacksonville · Ft. Myers · Sarasota

TOM WELSH

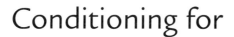

Conditioning for

Dancers

14   13   12   11   10   09   6   5   4   3   2   1

Library of Congress Cataloging-in-Publication Data
Welsh, Tom.
Conditioning for dancers/Tom Welsh.
p. cm.
Includes bibliographical references and index.
ISBN 978-0-8130-3390-7 (alk. paper)
1. Dance. 2. Physical fitness. 3. Kinesiology. 4. Dancing injuries—Prevention.
I. Title.
GV1589.W475 2009
792.89–dc22   2009019232

The University Press of Florida is the scholarly publishing agency for the State
University System of Florida, comprising Florida A&M University, Florida At-
lantic University, Florida Gulf Coast University, Florida International University,
Florida State University, New College of Florida, University of Central Florida,
University of Florida, University of North Florida, University of South Florida,
and University of West Florida.

University Press of Florida
15 Northwest 15th Street
Gainesville, FL 32611–2079
http://www.upf.com

My special thanks to the following individuals for their contributions to this work—

Photography: Rick McCullough; Whitney Earnhardt, assistant

Illustrations: Elizabeth Shanks

Dancers: Laura Beare, Kim Holt, Kehinde Ishangi, Maggie Cloud, Maxey Koch, Kit McDaniel, Chelsea Rodriguez, Philip Ancheta, and Jillian Vincent

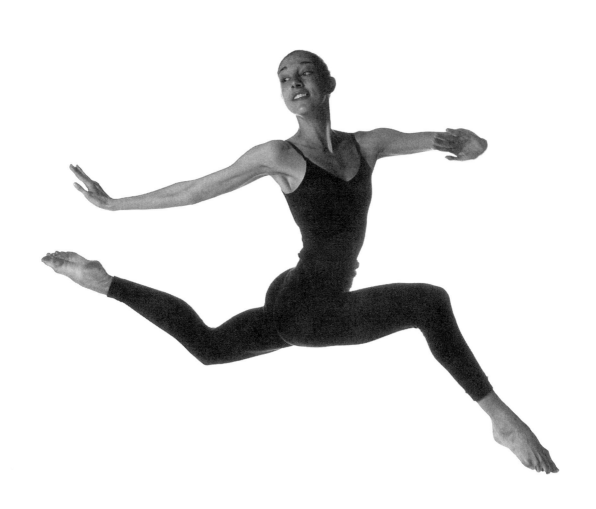

Contents

Introduction

This section gives background information that will help you understand the approach taken in the rest of the textbook, so please read it first.

Purpose

Conditioning for Dancers is a resource for dancers and other active people who approach training their bodies as carefully as professional dancers do. It describes the principles of physical conditioning in a manner designed to help all dancers apply the principles to their own training. It also identifies resources that dancers can use to build on the foundation that will be gained by reading the text.

Many fitness specialists recommend a comprehensive, single-system approach to fitness conditioning. Comprehensive training programs are ideal for individuals with the time and financial resources to pursue them. Many dancers, however, need a less comprehensive supplement to the system of training they are already receiving as dancers.

Conditioning for Dancers is designed to help dancers learn to play a more active role in directing their own training and development. Part 1 explains the concepts involved in physical conditioning. With a fundamental understanding of the physical capacities essential for dance and of the physiological principles that govern the development of those capacities, dancers will be better prepared to choose exercises and training approaches to match their current needs.

Parts 2 and 3 describe a variety of exercises useful to dancers and resources for learning more about them. The Resources section also offers a window into the variety of exercise systems that dancers may study more intensively when time and finances make such study feasible.

Probably the main contribution of *Conditioning for Dancers* is to distill existing information about physical conditioning into a form that will be immediately useful to busy dancers. I made a sincere effort to include only essential details. Dancers need advice on how to train, even in areas where the scientific basis for providing advice is imperfect and incomplete. I hope *Conditioning for Dancers* will be judged not by its scientific comprehensiveness but by its ability to help dancers improve their approach to training their bodies, the instruments of their art form. A delightful bonus would be for readers to seek additional information to expand and deepen their understanding of how the body works and how to train it.

My Teachers

Much of the information in *Conditioning for Dancers* came to me through the teaching and writing of others who train, treat, and conduct research with dancers. I have been particularly influenced by the work of Sally Fitt, Irene Dowd, Gigi Berardi, and Karen Clippinger. My hope is that *Conditioning for Dancers* will inspire you to study other teachers' work. References to many of the ideas in this text are identified in the reference list at the end of each chapter, and related materials are described in the Resources section. I tried to limit formal citations in part 1 to keep *Conditioning for Dancers* concise and easy to read. When you see an idea you want to learn more about, look for a related reference in the Resources section. If you cannot find the information you want, ask your teacher, fitness trainer, or physcical therapist for help.

Using the Text and Study Guides

Because I have condensed the ideas in *Conditioning for Dancers* to the fewest number of words needed to explain the concepts presented, most dancers will need to read it all to understand what is being said. Skimming or skipping sections will almost certainly compromise your understanding. Study guides are included so you can check whether you are understanding the main concepts. Any questions you cannot answer suggest areas you need to reread and think about more deeply.

One wasteful pattern some students fall into is copying another student's answers to the study questions. The practice compromises their understanding of the material and wastes their teacher's grading time. If you have not completed a study guide by a due date, admit your failing to your teacher and commit yourself to completing the reading and study questions as soon as possible. You may lose a few course points, but at least you will not miss the opportunity to learn concepts that may help you become a healthier dancer.

Acknowledgments

Conditioning for Dancers grew from a series of handouts designed to accompany brief lectures given at summer dance workshops. My goal was to present only what dancers absolutely needed to know. It was summer after all, and no one really wanted to be studying. Later, I began expanding the handouts into chapters, in part because the workshop dancers wanted to be able to review the information when they got home. My guiding principle was to use as few words as possible and to limit the presentation to the essence of each concept. The writing in these chapters has benefited from well-targeted feedback from first-year dancers at Florida State University and from dancers participating in summer dance workshops hosted by the Ballet West Conservatory and the Ririe-Woodbury Dance Company.

Several colleagues made contributions to *Conditioning for Dancers*. Mae Cleveland provided much of the detail in chapter 8, "Eating to Dance Well," which is based, in part, on a booklet for young dancers written by Andrea Jensen-Matich with help from Joan Benson. Margaret Wilson, Marjorie Moore, and Gayanne Grossman helped clarify many of the physiology, neurology, and injury concepts, and Laura Iverson and Elaine Durham Otto added precision and directness to the writing. Reactions by early reviewers Sally Fitt, Rachel Rist, Paulette Côté-Laurence, and Jim Costello were helpful in clarifying the audience and purpose for the text. Rick McCullough took the photographs with assistance from Whitney Earnhardt, and Elizabeth Shanks created the illustrations. Laura Beare, Kim Holt, Kit McDaniel, Maggie Cloud, Kehinde Ishangi, Maxey Koch, Chelsea Rodriguez, Jillian Vincent, and Philip Ancheta demonstrated the exercises shown in part 3 and the alignments shown in chapter 4. Sue Carpenter and many first-year dancers at Florida State University found typographical errors, missing words, and places of confusion so that they could be corrected. Melissa Croushorn handled the proofreading and Lila Sadkin created the index. New readers of *Conditioning for Dancers* will benefit from the efforts of these capable collaborators.

A Note to Scientists

Aspiring scientists may find the writing style used in this text too informal for research purposes. The text was written primarily for dancers who have little prior experience in applying science to their dance training. My goal is to introduce dancers to the benefits of a science-based approach by using familiar terminology and an informal communication style. As in a beginning dance technique class, new concepts are presented in elemental form to facilitate learning without distraction. Layers of complexity can be added to deepen understanding as dancers learn more about the dance sciences, just as dancers learn the complexities of turning and leaping as their technical abilities grow. This text is not intended as a model for science writing, but it does aim to provide useful information for dancers based on research conducted with dancers, athletes, and other relevant movers.

Suggestions Welcome

I hope you find *Conditioning for Dancers* interesting and that you discover creative ways to apply what you learn to your training as a dancer. If there are parts of the book that do not make sense or ideas that seem to conflict with your understanding of how your body works, please let me know what they are and where they occur so that I can correct them. Correspondence should be directed to:

Tom Welsh, Department of Dance
Florida State University
twelsh@dance.fsu.edu

PART 1

Dance Conditioning

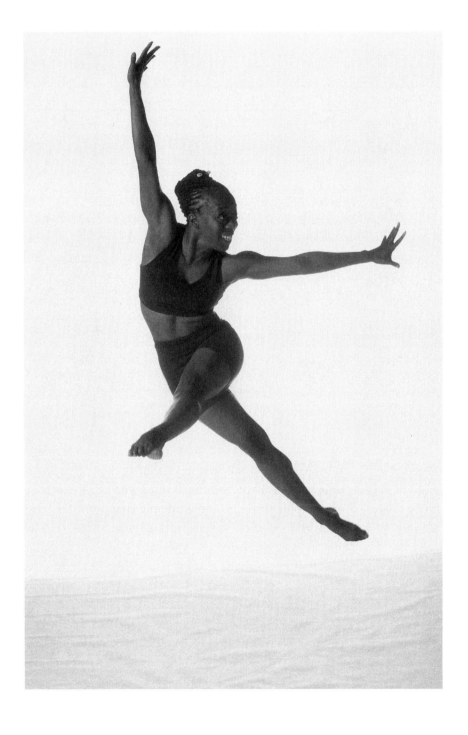

1

The Profession of Dance

Dance is a demanding profession. Full-time professionals can rehearse six to eight hours a day, perform eight or more times a week, and still take a daily technique class if they are lucky enough to be able to schedule and afford one (Berardi 2005, 9).

In addition to the tremendous volume of physical activity in the dancer's life, the variety of demands placed on the dancer's instrument—his or her own body—exceeds those of most physical activities. Dancers must be able to move with precision in ranges of motion that many human beings never experience. They must be strong enough to rise onto their toes and stay there, to leap into the air and land with grace, or to lift other dancers off the ground and return them safely and in time with the music. Dancers must be able to repeat these amazing feats as often as the choreography requires and to continue dancing through performances that can last an entire evening. To top it all off, dancers have to make everything they do look easy, and they have to look good doing it.

For dancers whose companies tour, the demands of traveling to new venues every few days, teaching master classes, and adapting to different theaters, climates, cuisines, cultures, and geography amplify the challenges they face. Professionals must learn to negotiate a truly amazing range of physical demands.

The life of the aspiring professional—the student dancer—is organized a little differently but is every bit as demanding. Performances may be more periodic, but the time saved from performing is filled with additional technique classes, choreographic projects, and academic class work for those who are still in school. Many student dancers work an outside job to pay for food, housing, and classes. If that work involves waiting tables, a common vocation for dancers, it places additional stress on their bodies. If dancers are to have a long career and not be crippled when they stop performing, they must manage the many physical demands on their instrument carefully.

Young dancers rely on their teachers (often a local studio owner, neighbor, or friend) and the resilience of their young bodies to negotiate the physical demands of training. As they commit to becoming professionals, as they begin working with teachers who are less familiar with their personal strengths and weaknesses, and as their bodies begin to settle into their adult forms, dancers need to learn how to take responsibility for directing their own training. Doing so can reduce the risk of injury, accelerate progress, and expand potential, thereby enhancing a dancer's career.

The purpose of *Conditioning for Dancers* is to provide dancers with tools for managing the physical demands they will face in their careers. Understanding the physical capacities that dancers need to optimize is an important first step.

Capacities Essential for Dance

There are seven physical capacities dancers need to develop to become and remain successful professionals. Most involve some physiological change in the dancer's body, but a few are primarily skill-oriented.

Alignment

Dancers must learn to align their bodies in ways that allow them to move efficiently. Performing multiple pirouettes or landing a *tour en l'air* usually becomes easier to perform once dancers improve their vertical alignment (Laws 2002).

Good alignment (sometimes called *placement*) can reduce stress to the joints and the muscles that control movement. Indeed, faulty alignment may be a frequent cause of dance injuries, and correcting alignment problems is usually part of the solution to chronic conditions such as tendonitis (Fitt 1996).

Efficient movement is important for making dancing look easy and for producing some of the subtle movement qualities sought by choreographers. Moving efficiently can conserve energy so that dancers will have a reserve to draw on when executing especially challenging skills or when performing the final sections in a lengthy performance.

Alignment involves *balancing on your bones* with just enough muscular engagement to sustain that balance with a minimum of effort. The task is complicated by the fact that what constitutes ideal alignment changes as the movement and the dancer's relationship to gravity changes. Good alignment is an ability to which all dancers aspire. Chapter 4 addresses this in some detail.

Strength

Muscular strength is the ability to lift an object (body, body part, or a prop) as high, as many times, and as fast as necessary. What we generally call strength is actually three related capacities: muscular strength, muscular endurance, and power. A set of examples will illustrate the differences.

Exercise physiologists define muscular strength as the maximum amount of force that a muscle or muscle group can generate (Wilmore and Costill 2004, 87). Strength can be measured in the laboratory, but dancers have a practical understanding of strength. The male dancer in a pas de deux, for example, must be able to lift his partner to the heights the choreographer wants. If he cannot lift his partner and return her safely and gracefully to the stage, he lacks sufficient strength and will have to build it gradually by applying the principles explained in chapter 2.

If the choreography calls for twelve lifts over the head, and the dancer can only do five lifts before tiring, he lacks sufficient muscular endurance. He might train this capacity by lifting his partner one more time each rehearsal (six times today, seven times next rehearsal, etc.) until he can lift his partner fifteen or more times in a row, to be sure he will have enough endurance to satisfy the choreography, even when tired or sick.

Power is a combination of force and speed. It involves being able to complete an effortful movement quickly. If the dancer can lift his partner the required twelve times, but cannot press her to the top of the lift on the beat, he lacks power. The dancer doing the lifting might train this aspect of strength by lifting his partner faster than the music—maybe even double time. There will probably come a point where the only way to increase his speed is to further increase the maximum force that his lifting muscles can exert (Wilmore and Costill 2004, 88). Muscular strength, that is, the maximum force that muscles can produce, appears to be the dominant component in this trio of capacities.

A well-conceived strengthening program will improve all three aspects of strength simultaneously. However, as the examples above reveal, sometimes an emphasis on one or another of the specific aspects of strength is needed. Training variety may be the best way to ensure that all three components of strength are being trained sufficiently for dance. Chapter 6 offers guidelines for increasing strength.

While the example above focused on strength required in the male dancer, female dancers know that the lifted partner often needs at least as much strength as her partner, although sometimes in different muscle groups. She has to be able to hold her body stable, in the sometimes evolving design intended by the choreographer, so that her center of gravity will remain over her partner's base of support (Laws 2002, 112) for as long as intended by the choreography. She has to be able to push herself off the floor hard enough and fast enough to help her partner lift her. She also has to be strong enough to catch and support herself as she is placed back on the floor and to make the transition imperceptible, even when her partner has miscalculated the lowering phase of a lift. In modern choreography, lifting roles are often unspecific to gender, and dancers are regularly called on to partner themselves as they move into and up from the floor. The development of strength is vital in the pursuit of a long, healthy dance career.

Aerobic Endurance

Muscles must have a continuous supply of oxygen to continue working. Oxygen is delivered to the muscles through the blood that is moved through the arteries and veins by the heart. Our lungs are responsible for putting fresh oxygen into the blood and pulling used gases, relatively high in carbon dioxide, out of the blood. Aerobic endurance involves the efficient operation of all these systems, and they all get trained during aerobic activity. Fitness trainers sometimes refer to this capacity as cardiorespiratory or cardiovascular endurance.

To improve aerobic endurance, an activity that uses lots of oxygen and pumps lots of blood must be continued for an extended period of time. Many dance activities do not train the aerobic system because they are stop-and-go, or intermittent, with rests between exercises and waiting in lines to cross the floor. Creative technique teachers can find ways to include aerobic activity in their classes, and a few dance science researchers are developing ways to make this easier (Wyon, Redding, Abt, Head, and Sharp 2003). However, even dancers who study with such teachers generally need additional aerobic training. Technique classes and rehearsals have other priorities and cannot provide all the aerobic training dancers need. Chapter 7 describes aerobic training strategies for dancers.

Relaxation

At first glance, relaxation may not seem like a physical capacity at all, or it may not seem important to dancers. But with a little reflection, dancers will see that the ability to release unnecessary muscular tension is key to efficient movement. Watch beginning dancers, and you will see excess tension in the hands, shoulders, face, and neck. Trained dancers learn to relax muscles not needed for specific movements. Selective relaxation of muscle groups is essential to achieving certain movement qualities, it leaves muscles fresh and ready to engage when they are needed, and it reduces unnecessary stress that can lead to overuse injuries. Like the other physical capacities, the ability to release unnecessary tension can be improved with training (Fitt 1996; Franklin 2004, 50). Chapter 7 discusses the topic of relaxation more in detail.

Body Composition

The final essential capacity for dancers is the ability to sustain a body size, shape, and look that satisfies their choreographer's intent. This is a capacity that I have alternately removed and reinstalled in this text. I take it out when dancers and teachers express concern that even mentioning it might encourage some dancers to develop an eating disorder. I put it back in because it is clearly important for dancers to find a productive way to address the complex challenge it presents.

It is obvious that in some forms of dance, long, lean bodies are preferred over all other body types. Dancers whose bodies are not naturally long and lean can get into trouble by trying to make their bodies match an image that is not realistic, given their genetic endowment. Happily, more and more choreographers seem to prefer dancers of different sizes and shapes, so devoted dancers whose body types do not fit one choreographer's aesthetic need only look a little further to find a place where they can be appreciated for what they can offer.

There are, of course, fitness and health limitations related to body composition. Being too lean, or too heavy, can jeopardize a dancer's health and career. If approached responsibly, however, maintaining a healthy body composition can work with the other capacities to help dancers optimize their potential and minimize injuries. Tools for finding the right balance are addressed in chapters 7 and 8.

Diversity of Demands

There are certainly athletic endeavors that require a higher level of ability in one or more of these capacities. Distance runners, for example, need greater muscular and aerobic endurance than dancers, and weightlifters need more power in certain muscle groups. However, there are few other professions that require such high levels of ability in so diverse a collection of capacities (Clippinger-Robertson 1988, 45). This fact was probably part of Martha Graham's motivation for calling the dancer "an athlete of God."

Summary

Dancers must optimize a number of physical capacities. They must be able to align their bodies and relax unneeded muscles to move efficiently. They must have the ability to move their bodies through extreme ranges of motion. They must have enough strength, muscular endurance, power, and coordination to make their movements precise and graceful. Dancers' cardiorespiratory systems must be able to deliver enough oxygen to sustain movement nearly indefinitely, and dancers must maintain a body shape that will get them cast. While other athletic activities require high levels of ability in one or a few capacities, dance requires high levels in them all. Optimizing these capacities can reduce the risk of injuries and limitations on performance. Learning how capacities change and grow is the focus of chapter 2.

References

Alter, Michael J. 2004. *The science of flexibility.* 3rd ed. Champaign, Ill.: Human Kinetics.

Avela, J., Kyrolainen, H., and Komi, P. V. 1999. Altered reflex sensitivity after repeated and prolonged passive muscle stretching. *Journal of Applied Physiology* 86 (4): 1283–91.

Berardi, Gigi. 2005. *Finding balance: Fitness and training for a lifetime in dance.* Pennington, N.Y.: Routledge.

Clippinger-Robertson, Karen. 1988. Principles of dance training. In Priscilla M. Clarkson and Margaret Skrinar, eds., *Science of dance training.* Champaign, Ill.: Human Kinetics.

Fitt, Sally S. 1996. *Dance kinesiology.* 2nd ed. New York: Schirmer.

Fowles, J. R., Sale, D. G., and MacDougall, J. D. 2000. Reduced strength after passive stretch of the human plantar flexors. *Journal of Applied Physiology* 89: 1179–88.

Franklin, Eric N. 2004. *Conditioning for dance: Training for peak performance in all dance forms.* Champaign, Ill.: Human Kinetics.

Graham, Martha. 1953. An athlete of god. Broadcast in radio series by Edward R. Murrow, *This I Believe;* rebroadcast by National Public Radio, Jan. 6, 2006.

Kimmerle, Marliese, and Paulette Côté-Laurence. 2003. *Teaching dance skills: A motor learning and development approach.* Andover, N.J.: J. Michael Ryan.

Laws, Kenneth. 2002. *Physics and the art of dance: Understanding movement.* Photographs by Martha Swope. New York: Oxford University Press.

Wilmore, Jack H., and David L. Costill. 2004. *Physiology of sport and exercise.* 3rd ed. Champaign, Ill.: Human Kinetics.

Wyon, Matthew, Emma Redding, Grant Abt, Andrew Head, and N. Craig Sharp. 2003. Development, reliability, and validity of a multistage dance-specific aerobic fitness test (DAFT). *Journal of Dance Medicine & Science* 7 (3): 80–84.

STUDY GUIDE

1. Briefly summarize the purpose of *Conditioning for Dancers.*

2. Why will most dancers need to read the entire text to understand the ideas it explains?

3. What are the seven physical capacities that a dancer must develop?

4. What makes dance an especially demanding physical activity, as compared with other athletic activities?

5. What benefits might dancers expect to receive by improving these capacities?

6. Do any of the capacities seem unimportant or unnecessary for dancers?

7. Which of the seven capacities is your greatest asset? Explain how you know.

8. Which of the seven capacities is your greatest challenge? What potential does it limit, and what risks does it present?

2

Principles of Conditioning

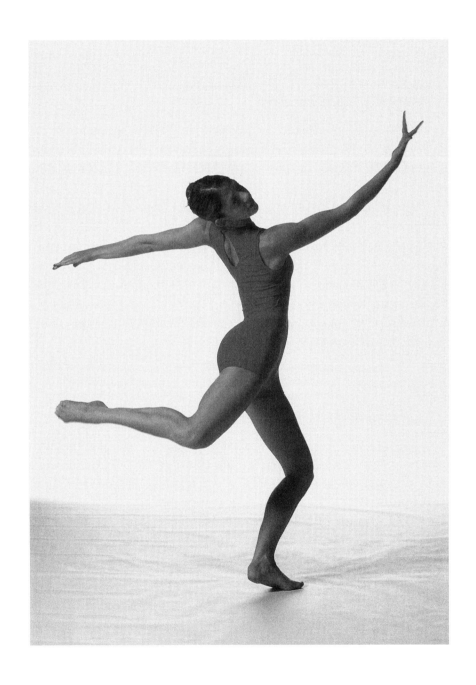

There are three principles, or laws, of physical conditioning that explain how the human body gains and loses physical capacities. They are as dependable as the law of gravity. Understanding them will help you figure out how to get the most out of your dance conditioning workouts. Understanding them will also help you recognize good conditioning programs and trainers and help you tailor training programs to fit your individual needs. The first and last principles have opposites, or corollaries, so there are five laws in all to remember.

Adaptation

When the human body is challenged repeatedly, it gradually develops the capacity to manage that challenge.

The first principle of physical conditioning, adaptation, explains how our bodies develop the ability to manage new challenges. Some exercise physiologists call this the overload principle (McArdle, Katch, and Katch 2006, 436).

The principle of adaptation makes it clear that we need to challenge our bodies to increase physical capacities (Alter 2004, 145). If we always work at a level that is comfortable, we cannot expand our abilities. Being uncomfortable some of the time is a natural part of the development process. Dancers and other athletes spend much of their training time pushing their bodies a little beyond what is comfortable; this is a necessary condition for improvement. When we challenge our bodies, they grow stronger. This is the principle of adaptation at work.

Reversibility

A capacity that is not challenged regularly will diminish.

Adaptation has a direct corollary called reversibility. If we stop working a trained capacity, that capacity will diminish or become weaker. Dancers experience the effects of the principle of reversibility when returning to class after a vacation. Some of the muscles that were trained to high levels before a break grow weaker with disuse and then get sore during the first week after returning from a break. Reversibility also shows its influence when dancers change teachers after working with one teacher for a while, especially if their teachers have different movement styles. The capacities unique to one teacher's training approach diminish while studying with other teachers.

In her textbook *Dance Kinesiology*, Sally Fitt (1996, 390) summarizes the principle of reversibility as "use it or lose it." When not challenged, our body loses its capacity to manage the challenge. This means that if we want to keep the capacities we need for dancing, we have to challenge them regularly. How often a capacity has to be challenged to retain its working level varies by capacity and by dancer. Some dancers seem to gain and retain strength with little effort but have to work daily to stay flexible. Other dancers do not seem to have a tight muscle anywhere in their bodies, but they have to work constantly to retain the strength needed to control movements. Approaches for maintaining various physical capacities are described in chapters 6 and 7. The key point is that you need to continue using the capacities you want to keep.

Specificity

Any increase in capacity will match the training challenge that produces it.

The second principle of conditioning is specificity. Specificity says that capacities expand to match the specific challenges our bodies face. Sometimes the specific nature of the training is obvious. Doing relevés, for example, will not make your arms and shoulders stronger, no matter how many you do, how much outside force you apply, or how often you train. To make our arms and shoulders stronger for dance, we must exercise them specifically, doing dancelike movements.

The principle of specificity applies to capacities as well as to movements. If, for example, you will need to be able to do 64 relevés in a row for a particular dance, your training should include doing lots of relevés in a row. If you need to hold your leg in high développé a la seconde for 20–30 seconds, you need to practice holding your leg in a properly aligned high second position, rather than doing battements through high second. Holding your leg using your hand might be useful as a first step to acquiring the range of motion needed, but you will need to practice holding high second with the muscles in your lower body to develop the capacity for développé à la seconde. The exercise needs to approximate (closely match) the specific ability you are trying to build. This makes designing exercises for dancers a craft.

Specificity also applies to the speed with which a movement is performed, the range through which the movement is performed, the body's relationship to gravity, and the movements that come before and after the movement being trained. So, for example, although the specifically relevant exercises for improving battement to the front will be similar to exercises for training développé to the front, specificity suggests that faster exercises will have more impact on battement while slower movements will have more impact on développé. In a Graham class, a contraction in a seated position and the first movement in pleadings (which begins lying supine on the floor) requires a different balance in the muscles used, even though the shape of the movements is similar. This is true because the influence of gravity is different when sitting than it is while lying on one's back. Finally, as any dancer can tell you, balancing after a simple plié-relevé is much different than balancing after a double pirouette. Practicing balancing after a variety of movements will make your balances more versatile. We need to match our training to the type of challenges we expect to face.

If we can identify all the aspects of a movement that need to be trained, we can design a specific exercise to gradually increase the ability to perform that movement. If, however, we do not know the exact movement, speed, range, quality, etc., that we will need to perform (which is often the case for dancers), varying training may be the best way to prepare. This suggests that, if you know you will only perform one choreographer's repertoire, you may do well studying one technique. However, if you expect to work with a variety of choreographers and teachers or dance in more than one style, you will need to vary your training.

In summary, if you can pinpoint a specific capacity you want to improve, try to design an exercise to match the movement you will be called on to perform. If you are not sure what demands you will face, develop and maintain a variety of capacities so you will not have far to go when presented with new challenges. There may still be an adaptation period, but a well-rounded dance instrument will adapt more quickly with less risk of injury (Clippinger-Robertson 1988, 76).

Progressive Overload

Our capacities expand fastest when the challenge is increased gradually.

The principle of adaptation explained the need to create a challenge to make our bodies grow, to work beyond our comfort zone. That challenge is called an overload. It is more than what our bodies are used to managing in terms of resistance, repetitions, duration, speed, or range of motion. The principle of progressive overload says that our capacities will expand fastest when the challenge is increased little by little, or progressively. We might, for example, do 20 relevés this week, 24 next week, 28 the week after, and so on until we reach the 64 relevés required for the repertory we will be performing later in the season. Increasing the challenge little by little is important for avoiding injuries (see chapter 3).

The principle of progressive overload can be hard to apply correctly. It requires patience and maturity to work gradually toward long-term goals rather than trying to become stronger or more flexible faster than our bodies can accommodate. The principle is also tricky to apply because the overload, or challenge, can be increased in many ways (Franklin 2004, 6–7). When building strength, for example, increasing the resistance just a little, the number of repetitions just a little, the number of sets by only one, and the number of workouts by one per week adds up to a sizable increase in overload, even though the change in each aspect of the dancer's workout is quite modest. It is the whole overload that must be increased progressively to optimize progress and avoid injury. Changing only one feature of the challenge each week would be a more effective approach. This makes it easier to see why it takes time to build new physical capacities. Learning to anticipate future challenges will improve our chances of being ready to face them safely.

Three guidelines for applying the principle of progressive overload include:

Working close to your current limits.
Moving with ideal dancer alignment.
Doing just a little more today than you were able to do perfectly yesterday.

The principle of progressive overload is like the law of gravity; there is no getting around it. You will develop capacities faster and safer by increasing the challenge little by little, day by day. Ignoring this principle will lead to problems that are explained by the corollary to progressive overload: compensation.

Compensation

Trying to progress too quickly invites bad habits and injuries.

Dancers know that if they try to work too far beyond their current abilities, they will compensate in some way, and this can become a bad habit that will have to be unlearned later. The tendency to compensate is a signal that the overload has progressed too quickly. If we do not back off when compensations appear, we might be injured. Progressive overload prevents compensation.

An interesting implication of this principle is that we need to *train the weakest capacities involved in a movement first.* For example, most dancers are strong enough in their hip flexors to do 50 or more sit-ups at one time. *[If you noticed that doing 50 sit-ups involves muscular endurance as well as strength, you are already applying what you are learning.]* Many dancers, however, find it challenging to hold the scooped-out position that trains the deep abdominal muscles (transversalis, pelvic floor, obliques, pyramidalis) long enough to complete that many repetitions. Dancers who do a lot of sit-ups without holding the scoop are focusing on their hip flexors and superficial abdominal muscles (rectus abdominis) and allowing their deeper abdominal muscles to stay lazy and weak. To build strength and muscular endurance in the deep muscles, roll up only as many times as you can while holding the scoop, then gradually increase the repetitions until you can do as many as needed without losing the scoop. For more about the abdominal muscles important to dancers, see Fitt (1996, 166–68) and Calais-Germaine (2007, 94–100).

Another example may be helpful, since this is such an important concept. The Pilates Reformer is an exercise device that allows dancers to adjust its spring resistance while training dance-specific movements. When working on the Reformer, many dancers can do pliés with all the springs attached; their hip, knee, and ankle extensors are strong enough to manage four or five springs. However, when starting Reformer training, many dancers cannot maintain ideal alignment at the pelvis and rib cage with more than a couple of springs attached. Maintaining ideal torso and pelvic alignment, while the legs are moving, is a less well developed capacity. Dancers often have to start with fewer springs than their legs can push so they can train their torso stabilizers to hold good alignment before they are ready to fully challenge the muscles of their legs. Approaching dance training in this way requires sensitivity, maturity, and probably some assistance from a skilled teacher or trainer at first.

To avoid compensation, we need to make efficient alignment and execution our top priority. We need to back off when we cannot maintain perfect alignment and execution, and we need to train our weakest capacities first. This approach will allow us to progress gradually and safely beyond our current limits.

Summary

The three principles of physical conditioning—adaptation, specificity, and progressive overload—and their two corollaries—reversibility and compensation—explain how the human body develops and maintains the capacities that dancers need to perform safely and effectively. It makes no sense to ignore them. By understanding these principles, dancers can optimize their development.

Principles of conditioning: How capacities develop

1. *Adaptation*—When challenged, body expands its capacities.
   → CHALLENGE your body to make it grow.
   Reversibility—When not challenged, body loses capacities.
   → Use the capacities you want to keep. (USE IT or LOSE IT!)
2. *Specificity*—Expanded capacities will match the challenges faced.
   → PINPOINT the specific ability you want to improve.
   Find or design an exercise to WORK that EXACT CAPACITY.
3. *Progressive Overload*—Capacities expand fastest and safest when the challenge increases gradually.
   → Start within your current limits; align and move perfectly.
   Do JUST A LITTLE MORE today than you did perfectly yesterday.
   Compensation—Working too far beyond current capacities invites bad habits and injuries.
   → Make PERFECT ALIGNMENT and EXECUTION your top priority.
   Back off if you cannot maintain perfect alignment and execution.
   Train the weakest capacity first.
   Use progressive overload.

You are now in a good position to fully appreciate this definition of conditioning by dance exercise physiologist Karen Clippinger (1988):

CONDITIONING

The systematic use of repetitive
and progressive exercises
to challenge key body systems.

References

Alter, Michael J. 2004. *The science of flexibility.* 3rd ed. Champaign, Ill.: Human Kinetics.

Calais-Germain, Blandine. 2007. *Anatomy of movement.* Seattle: Eastland Press.

Clippinger-Robertson, Karen. 1988. Principles of dance training. In P. M. Clarkson and M. Skrinar, eds., *Science of dance training,* 45–90. Champaign, Ill.: Human Kinetics.

Fitt, Sally S. 1996. *Dance kinesiology.* 2nd ed. New York: Schirmer.

Franklin, Eric N. 2004. *Conditioning for dance.* Champaign, Ill.: Human Kinetics.

McArdle, William D., Frank I. Katch, and Victor L. Katch. 2006. *Essentials of exercise physiology.* 3rd ed. Baltimore: Lippincott Williams and Wilkins.

STUDY GUIDE

1. Describe the three major principles of physical conditioning.

2. Describe the two corollary principles of conditioning.

3. How can understanding these principles facilitate your dance training?

4. What are the first clues that tell us when we are exceeding our current capacities and violating the principle of progressive overload?

5. What should we do when these clues first appear? What is likely to happen if we ignore them?

6. Why would it be difficult for dance teachers to apply the principles of physical conditioning with any precision in dance technique classes?

7. If the principles of conditioning cannot be applied with precision in technique class, what are the implications for training for a long, healthy career in dance?

3

Dance Injuries

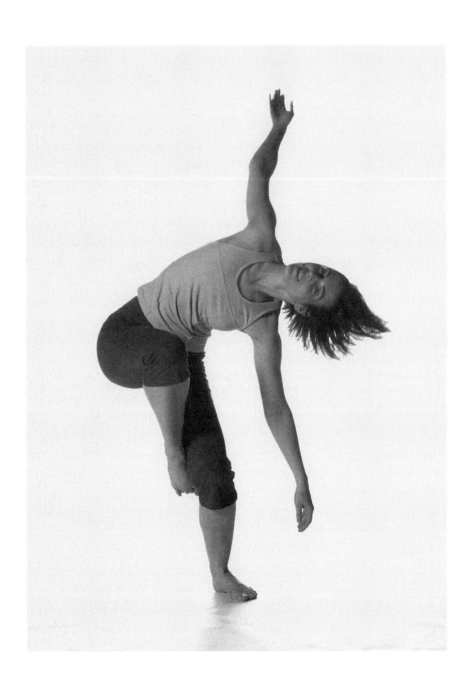

Dancers who have never had a serious injury can fall into the trap of assuming their bodies are indestructible, that they can never be injured. In her textbook, *Dance Kinesiology,* Sally Fitt (1996, 369) called this misconception the "indestructo phenomenon." It is not silly to assume we cannot be injured if we have never been injured. It is hard to respond to events that are not in our experience. Unfortunately, most dancers are at risk for injuries, not because they are weak but because dancing so often pushes the body to its limits. Understanding this risk may help you avoid injuries or at least minimize their seriousness.

Types of Injuries

One way of classifying injuries is according to how they first appear. Traumatic (also called *acute*) injuries appear suddenly, usually from a fall, a misstep, or an impact. A broken bone (or *fracture*) comes readily to mind when we think of traumatic injuries. A dancer who catches herself on her hands in a fall from some height may fracture her forearm. Dislocations are also traumatic injuries. They involve a disarticulation of a joint, and in dance they are most common at the kneecap (often called *subluxation*) and in the shoulder. *Sprains* result from moving a joint past its normal range, which can cause tearing of the soft tissues around the joint, particularly the ligaments that hold our bones together. When we pull a muscle, we have done damage to the muscle fibers or the tendons that connect them to the bone. If the damage is mild, it is called a muscle strain. If it is severe, it is called a *rupture*. Finally, a blow to the body can cause damage to the blood vessels and internal bleeding. This is called a bruise or *contusion*. A contusion in the head is called a *concussion* and is particularly dangerous because the rigid skull can cause the swelling to press inward on the brain.

While traumatic injuries occur all at once, *overuse* injuries build over time, usually owing to a weakness, faulty movement habits, or pushing the body too hard. Most dance injuries are of the overuse variety, and most of these injuries reveal themselves through inflammation. Inflammation is a combination of four symptoms: heat, redness, swelling, and pain. Probably the most common overuse injury for dancers is tendonitis, which involves inflammation of a tendon (the tissue that connects muscle to bone) and the tissues through which the tendon passes. Many dancers have experienced Achilles tendonitis or hip flexor tendonitis, because these are two muscle groups that are used intensively in dance. Bursitis and fasciitis are also overuse injuries that involve inflammation of other soft tissues like bursae,

Table 3.1 Injuries Common to Dancers

Traumatic	Overuse	Chronic
	Achilles tendonitis	Achilles tendonitis
Ankle sprain		Unstable/aching ankle
	Shoulder bursitis	Shoulder bursitis
5th metatarsal fracture	Peroneal tendonitis	Peroneal tendonitis
Ruptured disk	Low back pain (from fatigue)	Low back pain (spasm)

Note: Traumatic and overuse injuries can become chronic.

which are like ball-bearing pulleys that help tendons slide over bone, and fascia, the material that gives our muscles their shape.

The "itises" can be irritating and distracting. Their appearance is a signal for dancers to change the way they are working. Using a more efficient alignment or new pattern of movement or progressing more gradually may reduce or eliminate inflammation. Dancers who ignore an "itis" may be putting their bodies at risk for a stress fracture, which can be caused by repeated low-level stress instead of a single, intense impact. Stress fractures generally occur where the muscles used most intensively by dancers attach. Two common sites for stress fractures are the front of the tibia (shin) and the base of the fifth metatarsal (outside edge of the foot). Stress fractures can range from a hairline crack to crumbling of the bone under the attachment point for a muscle. Traumatic fractures usually heal rapidly and completely, as long as the dancer does not fall or get hit in the same way and as long as his or her nutrition is sufficient to build new bone tissue. In contrast, stress fractures can be harder to heal because the dancer must change the movement habits that produced the injury in the first place.

Both types of injuries, traumatic and overuse, can become chronic[1] (never ending) if they are ignored or if rehabilitation is incomplete. It is somewhat common, for example, for dancers and gymnasts to develop chronic Achilles tendonitis. At a minimum, chronic injuries distract dancers from their work as performing artists. They may also invite compensations that lead to other injuries or limit a dancer's potential. Chronic injuries can lead to stress fractures and other serious conditions, so helping injuries heal is essential for dancers. Before considering how dancers can help with the healing process, let's look briefly at the most common causes of dance injuries.

Injury Causes

The general cause of dance injuries is *exceeding our current capacities* either temporarily by a lot, as in a fall or impact that produces a traumatic injury, or by just a little but repeatedly (cumulative micro-trauma), which can become an overuse injury. Probably the major cause of exceeding our capacities is behavioral. Dancers who push themselves too hard, too long, too often, or too quickly set themselves up for injuries (Arnheim 1988, 3). As explained in chapter 2, we have to reach a little beyond our current capacities to grow; this activates the process of adaptation. However, pushing too much invites injury. Finding the right balance—learning to push hard enough to expand abilities, but not so hard as to invite injury—is the solution (Berardi 2005).

Faulty alignment and defective movement patterns are common causes of dance injuries. Both can cause mechanical stresses that seem unimportant at first but can accumulate to levels that cause injury over time (Clippinger-Robertson 1988). Correcting such problems before they become disabling is one productive approach.

Taking unreasonable risks in poor conditions also opens the door to injuries. Dancing at your limits on concrete surfaces or attempting your most challenging dance movements on slippery floors is unreasonably risky. Doing a maximum-effort run-though of a challenging dance after sitting for hours while lights are being set in a late-night technical rehearsal is also risky. If you have any hint the choreographer will want a full run at the end of a tech rehearsal, spend most of the tech time keeping your body warm, focusing on the body parts that are challenged most by the specific choreography. If you are surprised by a request for a run at the end of a long technical rehearsal, dance cleanly and precisely so the choreographer and lighting designer can see what they need to see, but stay in control to protect your instrument for the next performance and the rest of your career. Keeping your body healthy is in everyone's best interests.

Fatigue of the whole body or of a specific muscle group can also lead dancers to engage in injurious movement patterns. When your body is tired, it is harder for it to perform movements with the precision it knows how to use when it is fresh. Getting enough rest between classes, rehearsals, and performances will help your body use efficient alignment and healthy movement patterns.

Making new dances can create circumstances in which dancers unintentionally take unreasonable risks. When choreographers are trying to refine a new movement, sequence, or pattern in space or time (rhythm), they sometimes ask dancers to repeat a movement many times in a row. The choreographer is concentrating on the choreography and not feeling what the dancers are feeling in their bodies. If you are in such a situation and becoming so fatigued that you are putting your body at risk, it is reasonable to ask whether you can work on something else for a while. It is also reasonable to wear knee pads or shoes to protect body parts that are getting overused by repetition or imperfect execution when learning new movements. As you gain more experience with the movements and sequences, either your body will figure out how to perform them without additional protection, or your choreographer will realize that the choreography or costume must be changed. Alerting a choreographer to repetition fatigue and using the privilege responsibly will earn respect from choreographers and colleagues alike. It is in everyone's best interest for dancers to remain healthy.

Accidents also cause injuries, and they are preventable only some of the time. Minimizing the risk of accidents is, of course, a worthy endeavor. Preparing your body to handle unexpected challenges may also reduce your chances of injury. For example, developing extra strength in the muscles that control the ankle and foot may allow you to resist rolling over and spraining your ankle when you accidentally step onto a crooked foot. When an accident happens, review the circumstances to see if there is anything you can do to prevent a similar accident in the future. This is the only useful purpose for reviewing injury circumstances. Let the "If only . . ." thoughts go as soon as you have identified what you can do differently next time.

Nutritional deficiencies can also lead to injuries, both by weakening body structures and by depleting our bodies of the energy they need to give their best effort. Being properly fed is especially important when dancers are tired, distracted, or ill. Chapter 8 addresses eating to dance well.

Immediate Care for Dance Injuries

How an injury is treated right after it happens can have an impact on how quickly and thoroughly it heals. Because dance injuries often happen during rehearsals, classes, or performances, when medical professionals are not present, dancers and their choreographers and teachers are often responsible for immediate care. The acronym *RICER* can help dancers remember what to do when an injury occurs.

If you suspect any tissue damage, it is best to RICE the injury until the seriousness can be determined. RICE-ing a mild injury will cause no harm; failing to RICE a serious injury can make it worse.

Rest—The first step in caring for an injury is to get off the injured part to protect it from a possibly more serious injury. The expanded acronym PRICER is used by some to emphasize the protection component of good immediate care.[2] Dancing on an injured part of the body is likely to increase swelling and delay healing, and it may increase scarring. Sometimes the body is numb after an injury occurs, and the dancer cannot tell how serious it is. Staying off the injured part until you are sure it is safe to be on it is the responsible choice.

Ice—The second step is to cool the injured part, and this is usually done with ice. Icing will reduce swelling that accompanies damage to body tissues. Crushed ice conforms to your body's shape and makes better contact with the injured body part than cubes, but you will have to work with whatever is available. Having a sealable plastic bag in your dance bag and knowing where the closest source of ice is will be helpful when an injury occurs. If ice is not available, cold tap water can be run over an injured extremity. Water conducts heat dozens of times faster than air (Wilmore and Costill 2004, 310, 328), and since most tap water is much cooler than our body's temperature (98.6 degrees Fahrenheit, 37 Celsius), cold tap water (< 70 deg. F, 21 deg. C) is a reasonable substitute when ice is not available. Refreezable gel packs are a convenient source of cold because they do not leak their liquid contents onto bandages, clothing, and furniture. If you will be icing frequently, you might invest in a pair to keep in your freezer at home. With two, one can be freezing while the other one is in use.

Ice should not be placed directly against the skin for extended periods as it can damage skin and tissues beneath it. Different experts make different suggestions on duration, but a common recommendation is 20 minutes on and 20 minutes off. It is important to take the ice off periodically to let the blood flow freely through the injured limb to feed and cleanse the body tissues. Icing two to three times a day is the general recommendation. More usually will not hurt, and icing at least once is better than not icing at all. Do what you can, and do not allow failing to follow the guidelines perfectly keep you from trying to follow them at all.

Compression—Compression is the third component of immediate care for injuries. This involves squeezing the tissue around the injury just enough to keep it from swelling. Elastic compression bandages (such as Ace® or Tubigrip®) are designed for this purpose, so all dancers should carry one in their dance bag. A 3" by 5' (7 cm × 1.5 m) bandage is a good size for a variety of dance injuries. When wrapping an injured area, start a little further from the heart and wrap toward the heart to cover the injury, pulling the bandage just tight enough to cause a light squeeze. If you apply

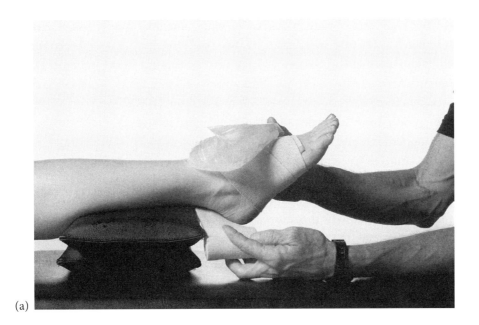

(a)

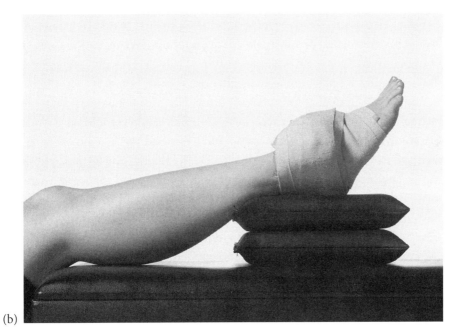

(b)

Figure 3.1. RICE-ing an ankle sprain (a) half wrapped and (b) finished.

the bandage immediately following an injury, the goal is only to prevent the injured part from getting any larger due to swelling. As with ice, the elastic bandage should be removed periodically to allow fresh blood to flow into the injured area to handle its cleansing and nourishing duties. There are some body parts, such as the patella, that should not be wrapped while exercising. Check with your health care provider to be sure.

Compression and icing can be combined by using the first half of the elastic bandage to compress the injured part, placing the ice directly over the injury, and using the rest of the bandage to hold the ice in place. This provides a layer of bandage to prevent skin damage, and it holds more of the ice in contact with the injured area. Also, by holding the ice in place with the bandage, the dancer can relax instead of having to balance the ice on the injured part. The bandage will insulate the injury from the ice for a few minutes, but soon the cold will penetrate the bandage.

Elevation—The fourth component is elevation. The ideal is to raise the site of the injury a little above the level of the heart to make it easier for the body to reabsorb any fluid that has pooled in the tissues surrounding an injury. This usually involves sitting or lying down with the injured part elevated. If an injury is in the ankle or wrist, elevation is relatively simple, even if it is not always comfortable. If the injury occurs closer to the center of the body, such as the lower back or hips, lying down will normally get the injury site close enough to the right level.

Referral—The final component of immediate care for dance injuries is referral for follow-up assessment, continuing care, and retraining.[3] Dance injuries, particularly acute injuries, should be assessed by a heath care professional to determine the degree of damage, to get advice on what activities can be continued without making your injury worse, and to receive treatment and a rehabilitation plan, if needed. Ready access to medical professionals who have experience assessing and treating dance injuries is a tremendous asset for dancers, schools, and companies.

> In case of injury . . . remember →   Rest
> Ice
> Compression
> Elevation
> Referral

Good immediate care for dance injuries provides two important benefits. It prevents an injury from becoming worse in the short run, and it initiates the process of complete healing. Knowing where to find ice, having a sealable plastic bag and compression bandage in your dance bag, and learning how to apply RICER are good preparation for the day when you or one of your dance colleagues sustains an injury.

Helping with Healing

Our bodies usually heal themselves if we let them. Unfortunately, in dance and other athletic activities, the (often self-imposed) pressure we feel to continue training and performing can make it difficult to give our bodies the stress-free time they need to heal. Dancers keep rehearsing to avoid getting behind in training or because a performance is coming up and they want to be ready. In addition, it can be painful to sit and watch class or rehearsal when we want to be dancing. There are a few things you can do to help with healing.

Continue RICE-ing until the swelling is gone. The minimum is usually two or three days, but if you are continuing to rehearse, take classes, or walk long distances to get to them, you may be causing new damage each day, and the swelling may continue for several weeks. As long as you continue to notice any of the indicators of inflammation (heat, redness, swelling, or pain), keep RICE-ing.

Heat can help with healing by increasing the blood flow to an injured area. However, *heat should be avoided until the swelling subsides* because heat can make swelling worse. Heat can help relax muscles and release cramping if there is no damage to the body tissues. Wet heat, like hot packs from a Hydroculator or a hot bath, will conduct heat more quickly than dry heat from a heating pad. Ultrasound is another means of creating heat. Ultrasound waves penetrate soft tissue and create heat when they reach denser tissue, like bone, essentially heating an injury from the inside out.

Some injuries require a judgment call to decide whether to use heat or ice. If you are fairly sure there is no tissue damage and fairly sure a muscle spasm is causing your pain, give heat a try. If heating the injury seems to make it worse, switch to ice. If you are just not sure, icing is the default until you can check with your health care provider.

Pain is your ally in the healing process (Fitt 1996, 370). Pain tells you how much is too much. When doctors believe the injured part of your body is ready to begin handling some stress, they often say to *do as much as you can tolerate without pain.* Masking injury-associated pain by using pain medications will remove some of the feedback you need to help with rehabilitation, so you may want to avoid taking pain-only medications if you can. Anti-inflammatory medications reduce all four components of inflammation, so they can actually facilitate healing.

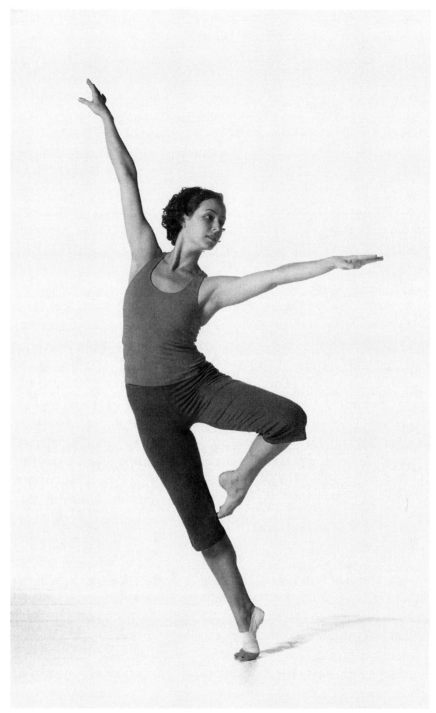

Figure 3.2. Taping a foot can facilitate the transition back to dancing following an injury.

Anti-inflammatory medications such as ibuprofen and aspirin reduce in-flammation, and there are circumstances that call for their use. Some danc-ers resist taking medications because they seem unnatural. However, taking anti-inflammatory medications when injured can reduce an irritation that might otherwise keep an injury site inflamed. Especially when advised by a physician who knows dance injuries, dancers should remain open to using anti-inflammatory medications as a temporary expedient. If you find your-self on a constant diet of pain medications, you may want to try correcting the underlying cause of the problem and save use of medications for when your body needs them most.

A key element of helping with healing is *selective rest*. Selective rest involves avoiding activities that irritate or put an injured part at risk of further damage. Athletic trainers and PTs (physical therapists in the U.S. and physiotherapists in other parts of the world) know a variety of *taping* techniques (also called strapping) that can be adapted for use by dancers to prevent over-movement and to protect an injured part of the body. To make the best use of this approach, look for a PT or athletic trainer who has expe-rience working with dancers. The range of motion dancers use is different from the range of motion used in other athletic activities. You will probably want to arrange to have the taping done just before your class, rehearsal, or performance, and expect to have it redone at least daily. Tape stretches, and if it gets loose enough to allow your injured body part to move too far, it will no longer protect the injured area from further damage.

Although taping can help, the most important component of selective rest is probably behavioral. You will want to *limit your activities to those that do no harm* to the injured part while *keeping the rest of your body as active as possible to minimize losses* in the capacities you will need when you are ready to begin dancing again. Get a clear description from your doctor, PT, or athletic trainer of which movements you should and should not be doing (including stretching, strengthening, proprioception exercises,[4] and dancing) to help with your recovery. Sharing this information with your technique teacher and rehearsal director before class or rehearsal can help by making unrealistic expectations, usually your own, less likely to push you to attempt something that may make your injury worse. The pain you experience with different movements will help you decide how much is too much. Keep reminding yourself that selective rest is temporary, and the better you are at keeping your exertion within the limits that your body can manage, the sooner you will be whole again and back to full participation.

A final aspect of being injured deserves mention. Being injured offers the opportunity to *work on a weakness* that you do not have time to address when you are healthy (Fitt 1996, 378). For example, if you have an ankle injury that keeps you from participating in ballet class, this can be a great time to work on upper body strength. The obvious advantage of seizing the opportunity is that when you return to dancing you will be more capable in an area where you were once limited. A less obvious but equally important benefit is that you will be playing an active role in your own healing, and that will make taking the time your body needs to heal more bearable.

When to See a Health Care Professional

Having an injury assessed by a health care professional is an important component of immediate care following acute injury. Dancers with easy access to professional health care should have acute injuries assessed as soon as possible to ensure that continuing to dance will not cause additional damage. Dancers who lack easy access to health care sometimes resist visiting a health care practitioner due to cost or concerns about time away from dancing. There are three general circumstances under which dancers should seek professional help with an injury, even if it is hard to get:

- You are worried you might make an injury worse;
- An injury is not getting better on its own;
- An injury keeps coming back.

Dance physical therapist Gayanne Grossman suggests adding these conditions to the list: limping or weight-bearing pain, inability to perform routine tasks such as reaching over head or running, deep pain, new pain, or pain that wakes you, significant swelling, or bruising. These conditions have potential consequences for the dancer's long-term health and career. Seeing a health care professional when faced with any of these circumstances is the responsible choice for yourself, your company, and your art form. Deciding whom to see may require some consideration.

Whom to See

Health care professionals have specialized training to address particular problems from a particular perspective. Dancers need to select someone who has the skills needed to address the type of problem they face. The approaches that dancers use to help with healing and to make their dance instruments more resilient range from those in which the dancer does most of the work while the practitioner educates, to those in which the practitioner implements a procedure and the dancer is relatively passive. Let's look at the range of professionals that dancers may see.

One group of professionals specializes in teaching efficient movement patterns. Some dancers see *Alexander* practitioners, who focus on alignment of the spine and the organization of movement around the spine. Dancers also work with *Feldenkrais* practitioners, who use exercises and gentle manual techniques to help dancers find more efficient movement habits. Specialists in the *Bartenieff Fundamentals* and *Laban Movement Analysis (LMA®)* teach more efficient movement patterns with help from developmental exercises. *Pilates* and *Gyrotonic®* trainers use specialized exercises and equipment to build strength and control in the center of the body to facilitate efficient movement of the limbs, particularly when using extreme ranges of motion.

Each of these movement education methods offers a different perspective on the challenge of teaching the human body how to move more efficiently. You may want to sample a variety of methods to help you decide which approach is most likely to suit your needs and temperament. Experience in several of these areas is probably useful for anyone who uses his or her body as intensively as dancers do. With this group of approaches, the dancer is correcting faulty movement habits with assistance from a teacher.

Practitioners in a second group do more work on the dancer's body, but may also engage dancers actively with exercises. *Massage therapists* release tension in the body with a variety of manual techniques. Some dancers include massage in their weekly training routines as a tension management tool. *Athletic trainers* also use massage but are even better known for taping (strapping) and for administering modalities such as ultrasound, hot packs, and contrast bath to encourage healing and to prevent injuries from becoming worse. Athletic trainers also guide dancers through rehabilitation exercises. PTs are usually trained to treat a wider variety of ailments, and they often design and supervise rehabilitation programs that athletic trainers implement.

A third group applies procedures designed to repair body tissues or correct imbalances, while the dancer generally has a much less active role. *Orthopaedic* and *sports medicine physicians* diagnose injuries, prescribe medications and physical therapy, set bones and apply casts, and do surgery. *Chiropractic physicians* realign the spine using manual techniques that range from so gentle as to be little more than suggestive to quite aggressive. *Oriental medicine practitioners* rebalance body systems using acupuncture, herbs, and diet.

What should be clear from this list is that, to heal and to stay healthy, dancers seek help from professionals with a variety of skills. Dancers have to choose professionals with skills to match their particular needs. So, for example, a dancer who experiences an acute injury that may have damaged body tissues will want to see a physician to get a diagnosis, a prescription, and, if needed, repair of any damaged tissue. In contrast, a dancer with muscle cramping that comes back whenever he takes a particular type of ballet class may want to begin by consulting a body work professional who is trained to look for and correct faulty movement patterns and imbalances that can lead to cramping. Of course, dancers can face a whole range of conditions between these extremes, and starting with one type of practitioner does not mean the other types cannot be helpful at some point in the recovery process.

An ideal arrangement for dancers is to have access to a clinic with a broad range of health care professionals from body work trainers to surgeons. Dance medicine clinics are available in many major metropolitan areas and are being established in more areas all the time (Hagins 2002). Clinics specializing in sports medicine can be nearly as helpful to dancers, particularly if their staffs have experience treating dance injuries. Having a continuum of health care professionals available means that injured dancers have access to a mix of treatment and training approaches that can be matched to their particular needs.

If you are not sure what type of help you need, you may find that a PT can help you clarify your needs. Most dance PTs work closely with orthopaedists and chiropractors and have a good idea what these professionals can do for dancers. They also have training and experience in a variety of treatment modalities. In addition, PTs are usually well connected in their health care communities and can refer you to experienced practitioners.

In many locations patients are permitted to visit a PT a limited number of times without a prescription from a physician. However, PTs may be reluctant to treat some injuries until they have a conclusive diagnosis, and many health insurance companies will not pay for therapy unless a physician has prescribed them. Dance companies and dance training centers would be wise to establish a continuing relationship with a PT who treats dancers so she or he can be consulted when a dancer is unsure which type of health care professional to see.

There once were stories of dancers being advised to just stay off an injury until it healed or to quit dance altogether (Fitt 1996, 368). As sports medicine has matured and medical practitioners have gained more experience with athletes pursuing professional careers, they have learned to design rehabilitation programs that keep athletes active. The same is beginning to happen in dance medicine, even outside major centers for dance. Finding health care providers who have experience working with dancers will give you confidence that you are getting the best care possible for your ailment.

When you visit health care professionals, particularly those who require less active involvement from their patients, be prepared to ask what you can do to help with healing. Many patients just want physicians to fix them, so your physician may initially be surprised by your questions. But she or he will respect you for wanting to do all you can. Working with a patient who is willing to invest significant time and effort in becoming healthier may be refreshing for your physician.

Health care practitioners use the language of their specialization because it provides an efficient way of communicating with their coworkers. Dancers serious about training need to learn the language of musculoskeletal anatomy so they can benefit from this same communication efficiency. However, if you do not understand something your health care provider says, say so. Write out your questions in advance and take a friend to help you muster the courage to ask questions. If you leave the clinic without getting an important question answered, call back and ask to speak to the head nurse. Often the nurse will know the answer or will ask the doctor immediately. Other times, the nurse will get an answer when the doctor is between patients and then call you back. You and your insurance company are paying for the physician's expertise, so do not let being shy or forgetful rob you of the information you need to help your body heal. Your health care providers want to help you, so let them know what you need.

Avoiding Injuries

Healing well from an injury is important to dancers, but it is even better to avoid injuries in the first place. There are several things dancers can do to reduce risks. Doing them will not guarantee an injury-free career, but it may make injuries less likely and less severe if they occur.

Perhaps the most important practice for avoiding dance injuries is to *warm up* before classes, rehearsals, and performances and to *cool down* when they are over (Alter 2004). Asking your body to do something it is not ready to do invites injury. When younger, dancers can sometimes get away with minimal warm-up and cooldown. but as bodies age, they become less forgiving.

Stretching your limits gradually, little by little (progressive overload), is another strategy. It takes about six weeks of focused effort to build new capacity, so start training well before you need to use it.

Build a reserve in all major capacities to draw on when needed. Having just enough strength to stand en pointe when your pirouette is perfectly balanced may not be enough to manage turns when you are slightly off-balance. Running a long and energetic dance more than once during a rehearsal is a good way to build an endurance reserve that might help you get through a performance safely when you are tired or sick. Look for ways to build a little extra capacity.

Movements repeated often can create strength or flexibility imbalances that invite injury. Finding ways to *create balanced strength and flexibility*[5] throughout the body is as important for dancers as it is for any athlete. This, of course is a primary purpose of adding supplemental conditioning to the dancer's daily routine.

Use caution in risky conditions such as performing on hard or slippery floors and performing when fatigued or not warm. Give the best performance you can under the circumstances, and save your fiercest efforts for better conditions.

Avoid bad pain. Sharp, focused pain usually indicates excessive stress to your body tissues. It is your body saying, "Stop whatever you are doing right now, or I am going to break." If you ignore these signals, your body will eventually break, and you will have to stop to repair it anyway.

There are milder, more generalized discomforts that dancers work with daily to expand their capabilities. The burning sensation that accompanies a movement that is repeated many times in a row and the tingling sensation that occurs when a muscle is being stretched are both indicators of work that leads to improvement. Wise dancers use these sensations to inform their training efforts. To learn more about good and bad pain, see chapter 18 in *Dance Kinesiology* (Fitt 1996).

Finally, *deal with problems* before they become serious. That irritation in your ankle, the tightness in your neck and shoulders, or your teacher's repeated reminders to keep your pelvis neutral during pliés and jumps are all signals to change something about how you are working. Ignoring such warnings invites injury (Wright 1985, 13).

Chapter Summary

Dancers regularly push their bodies to their physical limits, so many dancers will experience an injury at some time during their careers. The trick is to catch injuries before they become debilitating and to take action to minimize or eliminate their causes. RICE is the first course of action when an injury does occur. Choosing the right health care professional(s) and asking what you can do to help will expedite healing. Working on a weakness is a great way to make good use of injury recovery time. The best approach to injuries is to avoid them by minimizing risks.

Notes

1. The terms *overuse* and *chronic* are often used interchangeably, but the first addresses how an injury arises and the second indicates whether it stays around.

2. Margaret Wilson at the University of Wyoming suggests adding a *P* to get PRICER to emphasize protection when administering immediate care.

3. Rachel Rist at the Tring Arts Academy in the United Kingdom suggested adding "Referral" as the fifth step in the immediate care protocol.

4. Proprioception exercises are used by rehabilitation specialists to retrain the senses that coordinate reflexive movements essential for balance.

5. Gayanne Grossman at Temple University and Mullenburg College stresses the importance of creating balance in the dancer's body. Margaret Wilson made a similar point while reading chapter 1.

References

Alter, Michael J. 2004. *The science of flexibility.* 3rd ed. Champaign, Ill.: Human Kinetics.

Arnheim, Daniel D. 1988. *Dance injuries: Their prevention and care.* 2nd ed. Pennington, N.J.: Princeton Book Company.

Berardi, Gigi. 2005. *Finding balance: Fitness, training, and health for a lifetime in dance.* 2nd ed. New York: Routledge.

Clippinger-Robertson, Karen. 1988. Principles of dance training. In Priscilla M. Clarkson and Margaret Skrinar, eds., *Science of dance training,* 45–90. Champaign, Ill.: Human Kinetics.

Fitt, Sally S. 1996. *Dance kinesiology.* 2nd ed. New York: Schirmer.

Hagins, Marshall, ed. 2002. *Dance medicine resource guide.* 2nd ed. Andover, N.J.: J. Michael Ryan.

Wilmore, Jack H., and David L. Costill. 2004. *Physiology of sport and exercise.* 3rd ed. Champaign, Ill.: Human Kinetics.

Wright, Stuart. 1985. *Dancer's guide to injuries of the lower extremity: Diagnosis, treatment, and care.* New York: Cornwall Books.

STUDY GUIDE

1. What is the "indestructo phenomenon," and why are young dancers especially susceptible to it?

2. Explain the difference between traumatic and overuse injuries.

3. Give a dance example of each type of injury (bonus for examples not in the book):

    Traumatic

    Overuse

4. What does it mean when an injury becomes chronic?

5. What symptoms do the "itis" injuries have in common? (Hint: There are four symptoms and one summary term for the group of symptoms.)

6. What is the general cause of dance injuries?

7. Describe the five steps in providing immediate care for dance injuries.

8. If a dancer has just sprained her ankle and cannot get to ice, what can she do instead to satisfy the "Ice" step in providing immediate care?

9. Describe three things, in addition to RICE, that dancers can do to help with healing?

10. If you are not sure whether to heat or ice an injury, which should you do, and why?

11. When should you seek additional help from a health care practitioner to manage a dance injury?

12. Make a list of the types of health care professionals you would be willing to see if injured, and circle any you have seen in the past.

13. What is your greatest injury risk?

14. Based on what you learned while reading this chapter, describe one specific thing you can do this week to reduce this injury risk.

4

Alignment for Dancers

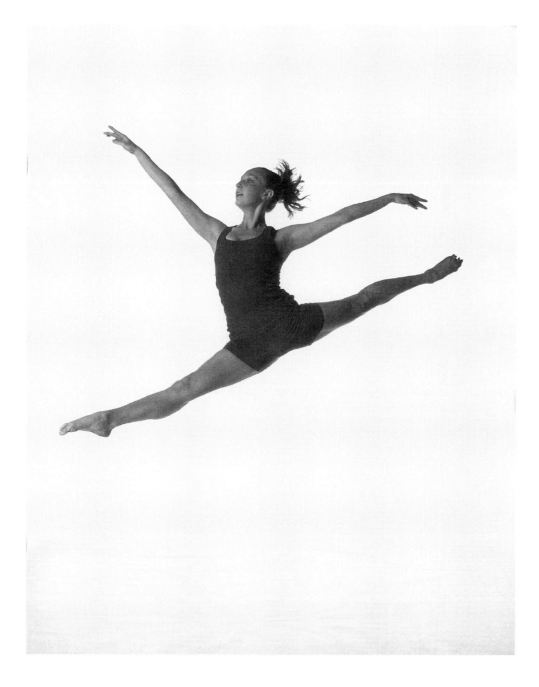

Experienced dancers know that good alignment (or placement) is essential. Good alignment makes our bodies feel and look longer, and it makes our movement more efficient. When bodies are in good alignment, standing is easier, joints work better, and injuries are reduced. Advice from anatomists, fitness trainers, technique teachers, and physicists who dance suggest that the most efficient alignments are those where the body is balancing on the bones like building blocks, rather than hanging from the muscles like a water skier hangs from the tow rope (Clippinger 2007, 30; Franklin 2004, 84; Grieg 1994, 26; Laws 2002, 20).

This chapter explains four biomechanically efficient alignments for dance:

1. Knees over centers of feet
2. Arches vertical
3. Front of pelvis vertical
4. Rib cage vertical over pelvis

These are not the only alignments important to dancers, but they offer a good start. Stylistic preferences may be layered on top of the foundation that these alignments create.

Each section begins with a description of one of the alignments and explains how to "see it" in yourself and other dancers. Being able to see good alignment from the outside is an important first step. After learning to see good alignment, you need to learn to feel it, too, so you can align your body while dancing without having to rely on teachers or mirrors. Each of the four key alignments has both "see it" and "feel it" cues. In some cases, descriptions of the two types of cues is similar, but in others they are quite different. If you have your own "feel it" cues that work for you, add them to the ones offered in this chapter so you will have several to choose from.

The photographs and diagrams are at least as important as the words, so spend some time studying them. To fully comprehend the essential aspects of this chapter, try out the alignments and the ways of seeing and feeling them on your own body as you read about them. That will make reading and studying a more active and satisfying experience.

Four Key Alignments

Knees over Centers of Feet

The first essential alignment is one most dancers have heard their teachers talk about since they began dancing. Whenever the knees flex, they should go directly over the feet. Because the knees and ankles are hinge joints, they flex most efficiently when they are not twisted. Most dancers can keep from twisting their knee and ankle joints by aiming their knees directly over the centers of their feet when doing pliés and when taking off and landing from jumps.[1] This alignment is better for the body whether the feet and knees are pointing forward in a parallel position or pointing more to the sides, as they are in the turned-out positions (1st, 2nd, 3rd, 4th, and 5th). This relationship is even correct when the legs are not in a symmetrical position, as in a lunge. Whatever the position of the legs, the centers of the knees should align with the centers of the feet so the ankle and knee joints can both hinge without twisting.

Some dancers mistake the direction their feet are pointing for turnout, and force their feet to point further to the sides than their knees can go. These dancers are pretending to have more turnout than they actually have. By trying to show more turnout than their hips can manage, they misalign their feet and stress their knee and ankle joints.

Dancers who force their feet to turn out further than their knees are probably using friction from the floor to hold their feet in an exaggerated position, rather than using their hip muscles to control the outward rotation of their hip joints. When this occurs, they allow their hip muscles to be lazy, and the principle of reversibility (chapter 2) takes over. What happens to these dancers' turnout muscles if friction from the floor is holding the turned-out position? What might happen if these dancers used their turnout muscles instead? The choice is yours, and so are the consequences.

After discussing proper alignment of the knees in a summer workshop I was teaching, I was surprised to see that many dancers' knees were still on a path that passed to the inside of their feet during turned-out pliés. When I asked, the dancers said they were trying to make their knees go over their feet, and they could tell that their knees were not going to the right place. It had not occurred to them that, if they could not outwardly rotate their hips enough to cause the knees to go over their feet, they could, instead, bring their feet under their knees.

There can be some confusion about when the knees are directly over the centers of the feet. For example, you have to be looking from straight above the knees to see the alignment accurately. However, most dancers can demonstrate correct alignment of the knees when asked to do so. They just don't use it consistently, and they put their knees, ankles, and feet at risk (Alter 2004, 151; Grossman, Krasnow, and Welsh 2005, 16; Negus, Hopper, and Briffa 2005; Vincent 1988, 103–4). See if you can identify good and poor knee-foot alignments in figs. 4.1a and 4.1b.

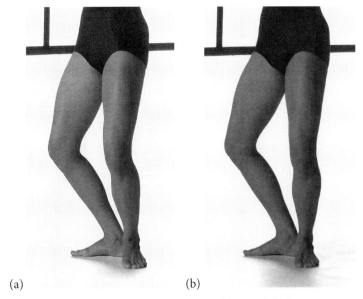

(a)   (b)

Figure 4.1. (a) Knees *not* over centers of feet and (b) knees over centers of feet.

> See it: centers of knees over centers of feet (in plié, looking straight
>   down)
> Feel it: knees over feet and feet under knees (feel it without looking)

The descriptions of the "see it" and "feel it" cues for alignment of the knees sound similar, but the senses used to detect good alignment are quite different. Now would be a great time to stand up and do a few pliés in first and second positions, pausing at the bottom of the plié to check the relationship of your knees and feet. Give special attention to how it feels when your knees are directly over the centers of your feet and how that feeling changes when they are not properly aligned.

Arches of Feet Vertical

Learning to see correct alignment at the foot is more difficult and requires some practice with feedback. The most sensitive indicator of good alignment is the relationship between three bony landmarks on the inside edge of the foot (fig. 4.2a). When all three landmarks are on the same vertical plane, like a window or door, foot alignment is ideal (fig. 4.2d). Good alignment allows the weight of the dancer's body to balance on the bones with less stress to the muscles, tendons, and ligaments, and it allows for shock absorption when landing from jumps. Good alignment at the feet can increase efficiency in the hips, knees, and ankles, as well as in the feet.

Two common misalignments at the foot are to let the top of the arch (landmark "B") fall inside or outside the other two landmarks. When the arch falls to the inside, the misalignment is called pronation or "rolling in" (fig. 4.2b). When it falls to the outside, the misalignment is called supination or "sickling" (fig. 4.2c). When we walk, run, or jump, some amount of pronation and supination are supposed to occur naturally to allow for shock absorption and efficient movement. Too much movement in either direction can create stresses that invite injury at the foot, ankle, and knee.

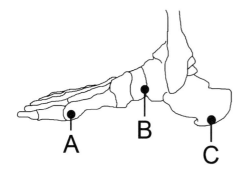

Left: Figure 4.2a. Alignment landmarks of the foot. A. Base of the big toe (1st metatarsal head); B. Top of the arch (navicular tuberosity); C. Heel (calcaneous).
Below: Figure 4.2b,c,d. Foot alignment using landmarks: (b) pronation, (c) supination, (d) neutral. Adapted from Fitt (1996, 37) by permission of Cengage Learning, Belmont, Calif.

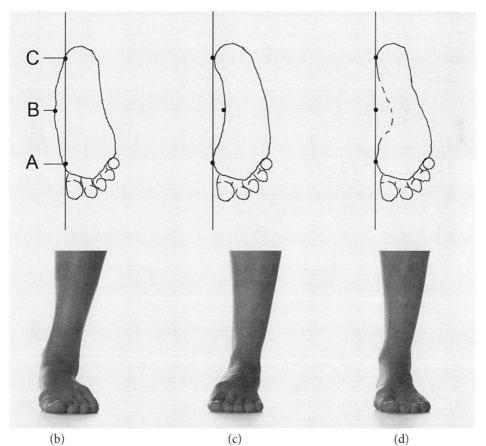

(b)   (c)   (d)

If you teach other dancers, a quick way to assess foot alignment is to look at the Achilles tendons. A parentheses shape (fig. 4.2f) indicates supination, and inside-out parentheses (fig. 4.2e) indicates pronation. When the foot is aligned properly, most dancers' Achilles tendons make straight lines (fig. 4.2g). Pronation is a common misalignment when the whole foot is on the floor (fig. 4.2e). It often accompanies misalignment of the knees (fig. 4.1a). These misalignments can put the insides of the knees and feet at risk. If you are experiencing pain in your knees, shins, or calves, check to see if you are overpronating, especially at the bottom of your plié or when trying to display maximum turnout.

Trying to lift the arches of the feet to vertical may irritate the muscles on the inside of the lower leg, including some of the muscles involved in shin splints. A better strategy relies on using three points on the bottom of the foot. Equalizing the pressure on the three points shown in fig. 4.2h will bring most dancers' feet close to ideal alignment (Gilbert, Gross, and Klug

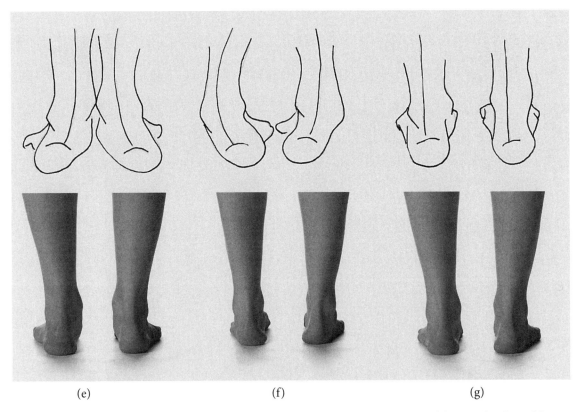

(e)   (f)   (g)

Figure 4.2e,f,g. Foot alignment using Achilles tendons: (e) pronation, (f) supination, (g) neutral. Adapted from Fitt (1996, 37) by permission of Cengage Learning, Belmont, Calif.

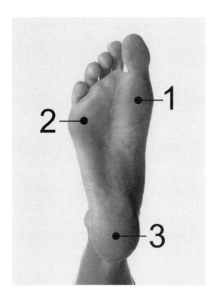

Figure 4.2h. "Feel it" landmarks on bottom of foot: (1) head of 1st metatarsal, (2) head of 5th metatarsal, (3) tuberosity of calcaneous.

1998, 340; Kravitz 1989, 599). This is a sensation dancers can use to assess their own foot alignment while dancing.

Feet See it: arches vertical; Achilles straight
       Feel it: equal pressure, three points on the bottom of the foot

Front of Pelvis Vertical

The pelvis is the point of connection between the lower extremities (legs and feet) and the torso. Good alignment at the pelvis is important for efficient movement. There are three planes on which pelvic alignment might be considered. Only alignment on the sagittal (front/back) plane will be addressed here.

For most dancers, the pelvis is well aligned when the top front corners of the pelvis (called ASIS, anterior superior iliac spines, or "headlights" by some dance teachers) and the lower front of the pelvis (pubic symphysis) are on the same vertical plane (fig. 4.3a and c; see also Kendall, McCreary, and Provance 1993). When the two ASISes are in front of the pubic symphysis, the pelvis is tipped forward, which is called *anterior tilt* (4.3b). When the ASISes are behind the pubic symphysis, the pelvis is tipped backward, which is called *posterior tilt* (4.3d). Posterior tilt is what some dancers call "tucking."

Initially, alignment of the pelvis is easier to see when lying supine (belly up) on the floor, which is a common starting position for many dance conditioning exercises. In this position, neutral alignment is when the three

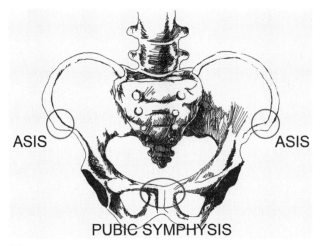

(a)

Left: Figure 4.3a. Pelvic alignment landmarks: ASIS—Anterior Superior Iliac Spines (*right and left*), pubic symphysis.
Below: Figure 4.3b,c,d. Pelvic alignment: (b) anterior tilt, (c) neutral, (d) posterior tilt. Adapted from Kendall et al. (1993, 20) by permission of Wolters Kluwer, Philadelphia.

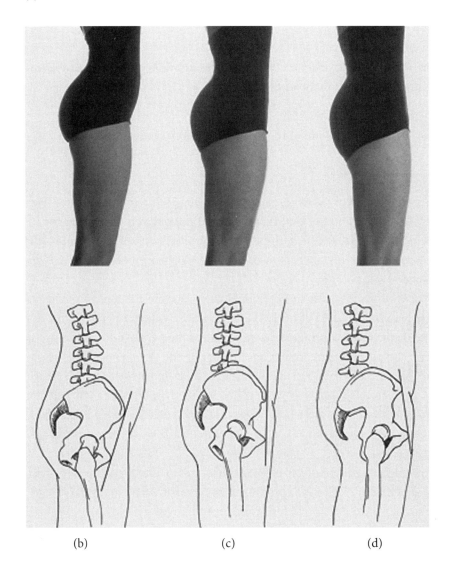

(b)   (c)   (d)

landmarks on the pelvis are the same distance from the floor, making your abdomen flat like the top of a table and parallel to the floor. A tea cup would balance on your abdomen when the pelvis is neutrally aligned. If your abdomen tips to spill the tea cup toward your feet, that is anterior tilt. If it tips to spill toward your head, that is posterior tilt.

Many beginning dancers allow their pelvises to fall into anterior tilt, which exaggerates the curve of hyperextension in their lower backs or lumbar spines (Calais-Germain 2007, 198). Some hyperextension in the lumbar spine is normal and healthy. Too much is called swayback or lumbar hyperlordosis (fig. 4.3b). Anterior tilting causes unnecessary stress to the lumbar spine, and it can shorten the muscles that cross the front of the hips. Anterior tilting can also compromise standing stability by putting the ligaments that stabilize the front of the hip joints on slack (Grossman et al. 2005, 17).

After receiving a little dance training, some new dancers learn to tilt their pelvises posteriorly, removing even the normal, healthy curve in their lumbar spines (Calais-Germain 2007, 198). New dancers probably make this overcorrection because it feels like they are working harder and it shows they are trying. But this misalignment can overactivate the quadriceps (thigh muscles) and gluteal muscles (tush), and may cause these muscles to become larger than necessary (Fitt 1996, 162). At the very least, the posterior tilting makes it harder to move freely.

One mistake that is easy to make when assessing pelvic alignment is to be distracted by body contour. Figs. 4.3e and 4.3f show how body contour can create the illusion of excessive lumbar lordosis when alignment of the spine (and pelvis, not shown) is actually correct in both drawings. The relationship between the ASISes and pubic symphysis is a more accurate indicator of pelvic alignment than body contour. Dancers can benefit from learning to use these landmarks to assess alignment in this area of the body.

Engaging the abdominal muscles can prevent anterior pelvic tilt, but engaging them too much can cause posterior tilt. A more sensitive cue is available to guide pelvic alignment. If you allow your pelvis to move freely between anterior and posterior tilt, you can learn to feel when the pelvis is passing the point where it is tallest and balancing on the tops of the thigh bones (heads of the femurs). Using this sensation as a cue for neutral alignment will encourage you not to lock your body into a position but, instead, to continually test your alignment and make small adjustments to keep the bones in balance and your body moving efficiently. This cue can help danc-

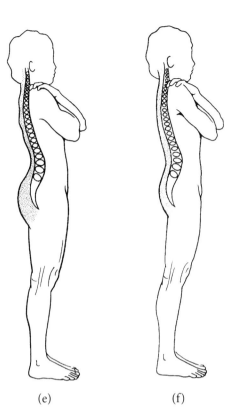

Figure 4.3e,f. Body contour can be misleading when assessing alignment at the pelvis and spine. Adapted from Calais-Germain (2007, 35) by permission of Eastland Press, Seattle.

(e)   (f)

ers find neutral alignment quickly on the Pilates Reformer without a trainer trying to steer them into a position that looks right from the outside.

Pelvis   See it: front of pelvis vertical
          Feel it: balance pelvis on heads of femurs

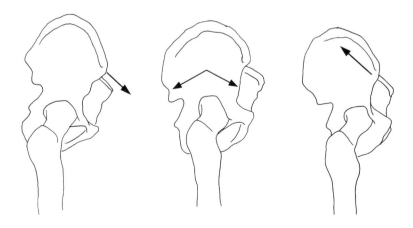

Rib Cage Vertical above Pelvis

The fourth alignment essential for dancers involves the relationship of the rib cage to the pelvis. When aligned efficiently, the rib cage is vertical and directly above the pelvis (fig. 4.4c). A common misalignment for beginners, and even for some experienced dancers, is to lift the bottom of the rib cage forward and up, which tilts the top of the rib cage back. This often occurs with anterior tilt of the pelvis (fig. 4.4a).

Lifting the rib cage forward may be another way of compensating for anterior pelvic tilt (Gamboian, Chatfield, Woollacott, Barr, and Klug 1999, 12). If you are tilting your pelvis forward, you can compensate by arching your lumbar spine (4.3b) or by arching a little higher in the spine (4.4a). Either will bring your head and shoulders to vertical.

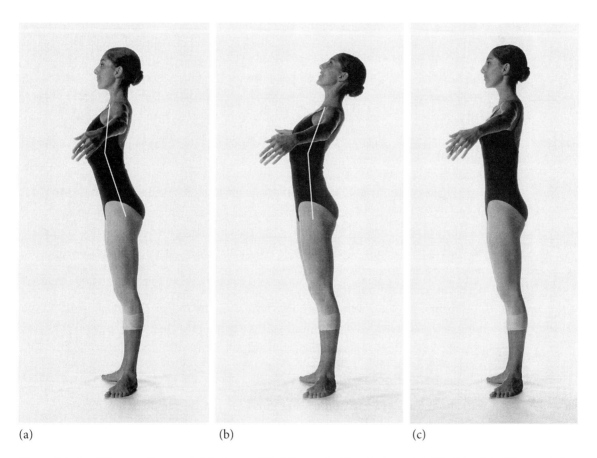

(a) (b) (c)

Figure 4.4a,b,c. Rib cage alignment: (a) rib cage lifted forward with anterior pelvic tilt, (b) pelvic tilt corrected without correcting misaligned rib cage, (c) neutral.

Other reasons for tipping the rib cage up and forward probably include overcorrecting slumping by applying the instruction to "pull up" to the wrong part of the body (Watkins et al. 1990, 171), and signaling readiness to dance by adding tension in a way that distorts alignment. Such patterns may be learned when dancers are young, and they become habits that get harder to change the longer they are used.

If pelvic alignment is corrected, misalignment of the rib cage is easier to see and feel. For example, if the dancer in figure 4.4a brought her pelvis to vertical without changing the bend in the middle of her back, she would be leaning backward (fig. 4.4b). Some dancers may resist correcting pelvic alignment because it makes them lean backward, and they know that cannot be right. Of course, these dancers are confusing the source of the problem and keeping one faulty alignment (at the pelvis) to cover up another (at the rib cage).

If the rib cage is always tilted, the muscles on the back of the spine will become shorter, making it more difficult to bring the spine into neutral alignment. When dancers with this habit try to flex their spines by rolling down to the front, they may feel pinching in the area where the muscles have become too short and may overflex adjacent parts of their spines to compensate. Like many misalignments, tipping the rib cage reduces movement efficiency and compromises the visual aesthetics of sound alignment. Take another look at figures 4.4a–c. In which image(s) does the dancer look the longest, most balanced, and most at ease?

Balanced use of the abdominal and back muscles can influence rib cage alignment. One way to cue better alignment at the rib cage is to have a teacher or partner place two fingers on the bottom, front corners of your rib cage and two fingers on the top back corners of your pelvis (posterior superior iliac spines), and try to bring all four of these points together in the center of your body (fig. 4.4d).

Dancers who rely solely on pulling with the abdominal muscles may create excess tension that will limit healthy motion in the spine, and they may even find it difficult to breathe. Making room for the downward and inward movement of the bottom of the rib cage by relaxing the muscles in the middle of the back and imagining the top of the sternum reaching forward and up can invite good alignment of the rib cage with less excess tension. Relaxing overactive back muscles will be easier if they are long enough to allow the rib cage to move into neutral alignment. So stretching the muscles of the spine will help if this is an alignment you have difficulty achieving. Try the upper spine → whole spine stretch (exercise 9) and the kneeling back stretch (exercise 18) in part 2.

Rib cage   See it: rib cage vertical, above pelvis
            Feel it: four points together in center of body

The fifth key alignment would be balancing the head on top of the spine. If you have achieved the other four key alignments, this alignment may take care of itself. If it does not, see if you can create "see it" and "feel it" cues for aligning your head on your spine. Alexander technique focuses on alignment of the head and how it influences alignment in the rest of the body (see Resources, part 3).

Alignment Interactions

The interactive nature of alignment of the rib cage and pelvis, as explained above and shown in the photographs, has implications for changing these misalignments. If a dancer were to align her rib cage with the pelvis without correcting an anterior pelvic tilt, she would tend to fall forward (fig. 4.4a). If the same dancer were to correct anterior pelvic tilt without changing the relationship of the rib cage to the lower back, the dancer would tend to

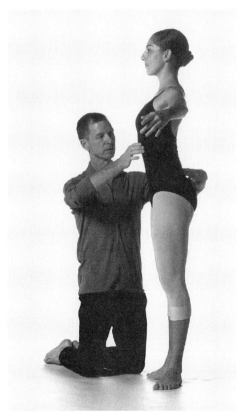

Figure 4.4d. Cue for correcting rib cage alignment.

fall backward (fig. 4.4b). Adjusting the two misalignments gradually and simultaneously toward neutral is likely to be the most effective strategy. In fact, this may be the strategy of choice for correcting many misalignments.

Tools for Improving Alignment

The four alignments described in this chapter—knees over toes, arches vertical, front of pelvis vertical, and rib cage vertical over the pelvis—can influence movement efficiency, aesthetic line, and injury risk. The rest of the chapter offers suggestions for what you can do to improve alignment.

Awareness, the focus of this chapter so far, is one tool dancers can use to improve alignment. Three others are *strengthening* and activating muscles that maintain good alignment, *stretching* muscles that prevent good alignment, and *relaxing* muscles that create unnecessary tension or compensations. The tools are complementary, so a balanced use of all of them will probably lead to the quickest and longest lasting improvements. For some dancers and some alignment corrections, using all of these tools may be necessary to achieve meaningful improvements.

Learning to describe and *see* the key alignments creates awareness that is an important first step in improving dancer alignment. Learning to *feel* the alignments in your own body further expands awareness and makes it possible to detect and adjust alignment, even while dancing. Two additional awareness steps can help dancers improve alignment. One involves *cueing* correct alignment when opportunities are presented. Another is *acknowledging* good alignment when you see or feel it.

Dancers can cue their own alignment by silently reminding themselves of the "feel it" cues while dancing. Sports psychologist Garry Martin and his colleagues (e.g., Ming and Martin 1996) have demonstrated the effectiveness of using self-cueing techniques with elite figure skaters. There is no reason why this approach could not work with dancers. In fact, many dancers already cue themselves much of the time while dancing, particularly during technique classes. If you teach other dancers, you can help them develop alignment awareness by teaching them the "feel it" cues and by giving the cues when there are opportunities to use the alignments in class.

Acknowledging success is also important, especially when starting to make a change. Any change in alignment is likely to feel wrong at first, so you may have to remind yourself that the new alignment is more efficient even if it feels strange. As your body becomes more familiar with new alignments, and you begin to experience the benefits they produce, they will begin to feel right, and extra cueing may become unnecessary.

Let's see how these strategies might be used to improve alignment of the pelvis. You might begin by learning to see the ideal relationship between the landmarks (2 ASISes and pubic symphysis) and by practicing *seeing* when other dancers' pelvises are neutrally aligned while lying supine and while standing at the barre. You might also learn to *feel* your own pelvis balancing on the heads of your femurs while standing and while working supine on the Pilates Reformer. You might refine your alignment awareness by rocking your pelvis forward and backward to learn to feel the neutral point while bridging (exercise 15), and while finding neutral alignment from various misaligned standing positions. You might try doing pliés with anterior tilt, posterior tilt, and neutral alignment to become more aware of the differences. You might silently remind yourself to "balance the pelvis on the heads of the femurs" while you are at the barre and acknowledge your own success in doing so after each exercise. As awareness improves and your natural style of self-monitoring takes over, you will probably find you can give less attention to cueing and assessment.

Building the refined strength needed to maintain good alignment is another useful tool that can be added to improve awareness. Exercises to *strengthen* muscles that can help dancers balance their pelvis on their femurs (deep abdominal and back muscles, pelvic floor, and hamstrings) might be repeated to fatigue every day until you have enough strength in these muscle groups to bring your pelvis into balance while dancing. In addition to neutral bridging (exercise 15), other strengthening exercises that emphasize neutral pelvic alignment are torso/pelvis stabilization (exercise 14), tendue arabesque prone (exercise 16), and plank support (exercise 19). How much strength is enough will depend on the choreography you are likely to face. Once sufficient strength is gained, a maintenance program will normally be needed to retain strength (see chapter 6).

A common inhibitor of ideal alignment at the pelvis is short (tight) hip flexors. A *stretching* program for the hip flexors including kneeling lunge, TV stretch, and their variations (exercise 23) can make it easier to achieve and maintain good pelvic alignment. Increasing the length of the hip flexors reduces the work required from the muscles that hold good pelvic alignment—a complementary effect. Back stretches (exercises 8 and 18) can also make it easier to achieve good alignment at the pelvis.

Many dancers find their alignment benefits from learning to *relax* the muscles that interfere with good pelvic alignment. Overactive hip flexors and lower back extensors can tip the pelvis forward, and overactive quadriceps and gluteal muscles can make it hard to move freely. A targeted re-laxation exercise such as hip lift (exercise 30) can help you develop the ability to release unnecessary tension (see also Fitt 1996, 432). Progressive relaxation (see chapter 7) can also help, particularly for dancers who have little or no experience with tension releasing exercises. Of course, relax-ation is an oversimplification. If you relaxed completely, you would end up in a puddle on the floor. What is needed for proper alignment and efficient movement is just enough engagement, of just the right muscles, at just the right time, in just the right pattern. This is an issue of neuromuscular coor-dination that is a training priority in technique classes and in many of the somatic training techniques (see part 3 for resources).

> *See, feel, cue, acknowledge* good alignment (awareness)
> *Strengthen* muscles that maintain good alignment
> *Stretch* muscles that prevent good alignment
> *Relax* muscles that do the wrong thing

Summary

The four tools of awareness, strengthening, stretching, and relaxing can help dancers improve alignment. This can help dancers move more effi-ciently, increase movement potential, and reduce injury risk. In this chap-ter, we looked at awareness in some detail. Chapters 6 and 7 will offer more detail on improving strength, flexibility, and the ability to release unneces-sary tension.

Note

1. While most dancers' knee and ankle joints are the least twisted when the knees go over the centers of the feet, this is not true for every dancer. For dancers who have a fair amount of twist in their shins (tibial torsion), the knee and ankle joints never align perfectly because the bending axes for the knees and ankles are at different angles. This means any time the knees and ankles flex at the same time (and that happens a lot in dance), there is probably some twisting in the joints. For dancers with tibial torsion, the goal is to find a relationship between the knee and foot that minimizes stress on the joints. If tibial torsion is a challenge you face, ask your dance teacher, fitness trainer, or PT to help you find a good compromise for your body. If you are borderline, or not sure, try for knees over feet for a while, and if it is not working, seek help. To learn more about tibial torsion in dancers, see Grossman et al. (2008).

References

Alter, Michael J. 2004. *The science of flexibility.* 3rd ed. Champaign, Ill.: Human Kinetics.

Calais-Germain, Blandine. 2007. *Anatomy of movement.* Seattle: Eastland.

Clippinger, Karen. 2007. *Dance anatomy and kinesiology.* Champaign, Ill.: Human Kinetics.

Fitt, Sally S. 1996. *Dance kinesiology.* 2nd ed. New York: Schirmer.

Franklin, Eric N. 2004. *Conditioning for dance: Training for peak performance in all dance forms.* Champaign, Ill.: Human Kinetics.

Gamboian, N., S. J. Chatfield, M. H. Woollacott, S. Barr, and G. A. Klug. 1999. Effects of dance technique training and somatic training on pelvic tilt and lumbar lordosis alignment during quiet stance and dynamic dance movement. *Journal of Dance Medicine & Science* 3 (1): 7–14.

Gilbert, Coryleen B., Michael T. Gross, and Kimberly B. Klug. 1998. Relationship between hip external rotation and turnout angle for the five classical ballet positions. *Journal of Orthopaedic & Sports Physical Therapy* 27 (5): 339–47.

Grieg, Valerie. 1994. *Inside ballet technique: Separating anatomical fact from fiction in the ballet class.* Pennington, N.J.: Princeton Book Company.

Grossman, Gayanne, Donna Krasnow, and Tom Welsh. 2005. Effective use of turnout: Biomechanical, neuromuscular, and behavioral considerations. *Journal of Dance Education* 5: 15–27.

Grossman, Gayanne, K. N. Waninger, A. Volshin, W. R. Reinus, R. Ross, J. Stoltzfus, and K. Bibalo. 2008. Reliability and validity of goniometric turnout measurements compared with MRI and retro-reflective markers. *Journal of Dance Medicine & Science* 12 (4): 142–52.

Kendall, Florence P., Elizabeth K. McCreary, and Patricia G. Provance. 1993. *Muscle testing and function.* 4th ed. Baltimore: Williams and Wilkins.

Kravitz, Steven R. 1989. The mechanics of dance and dancer related injuries. In Steven I. Subotnick, ed., *Sports medicine of the lower extremity,* 595–603. New York: Churchill Livingstone.

Laws, Kenneth. 2002. *Physics and the art of dance.* Oxford: Oxford University Press.

Ming, S., and G. Martin. 1996. Single-subject evaluation of a self-talk package for improving figure skating performance. *Sport Psychologist* 10: 227–38.

Negus, Vicki, Diana Hopper, and N. Kathryn Briffa. 2005. Associations between turnout and lower extremity injuries in classical ballet dancers. *Journal of Orthopaedic & Sports Physical Therapy* 35 (5): 307–18.

Vincent, Larry M. 1988. *The dancer's book of health.* Hightstown, N.J.: Princeton Book Company.

Watkins, Andrea, and Priscilla M. Clarkson. 1990. *Dancing longer, dancing stronger: A dancer's guide to improving technique and preventing injury.* Princeton, N.J.: Princeton Book Company.

STUDY GUIDE

1. What four alignments are essential for dancers?

2. What benefits can dancers expect to receive as they get closer to the ideal in each of these alignments?

3. List the "feel it" cues for each of the key alignments. If you have a different cue that works for you while dancing, add it as an extra cue to the list.

4. What is the quickest way for teachers to see if a dancer's foot is close to neutral alignment?

5. What misalignment of the pelvis is common for beginning dancers? Why might this misalignment be common in beginners?

6. What misalignment of the pelvis do dancers learn to perform after they have had some dance training? Why would dancers adopt this new misalignment?

7. Briefly explain four tools that dancers can use to correct misalignments.

8. Which tool do you think is most important? Why?

9. Which of the key alignments do you have the most room to improve? How do you know?

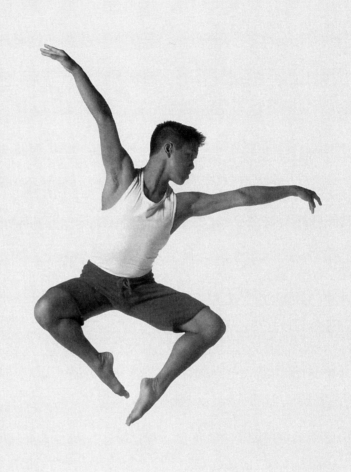

5

Warm-up and Cooldown

Before addressing how to improve specific physical capacities in chapters 6 and 7, this chapter will address the warm-up and cooldown. Experienced dancers and teachers often advocate warming-up at the beginning of every dance class, rehearsal, and performance and cooling down when the activity ends. Technique classes often include a warm-up as an integral part of the lesson (White 1996, 130). Cooldowns are less universal, but are included in some technique classes. For other studio classes and rehearsals, the warm-up and cooldown are usually left to the dancer.

If you are certain your teacher or rehearsal director will include a warm-up in your class or rehearsal, you may only need to supplement the class warm-up with any special preparation you know your body will need. If you are not sure whether a sufficient warm-up will be given, or if you want to be at your best from the start of class, then doing your own warm-up before your class or rehearsal begins is the best practice.

Cooldown comes after dancing, so you can determine what your body needs when each class, rehearsal, or performance ends. The challenge with cooldown is not about anticipating your needs in advance but about resisting the temptation to do something else before you finish a cooldown. Let's take a closer look at the warm-up and cooldown and consider what you may do to ensure your body is getting what it needs.

Warm-up

Why warm up? The human body is, among other things, a biomechanical system designed for movement. All mechanical systems, even your car, work better after they are warmed up. In fact, attempting to operate mechanical systems at peak levels without warm-up can make them susceptible to damage. If you were to push your car's accelerator to the floor right after you started it on a cold winter morning, you might cause serious damage to the engine. Biomechanical systems, like the human musculoskeletal system, are at least as vulnerable if not warmed up. As with your car, you may not see the damage immediately, but it will catch up with you eventually. Unlike your car, you cannot go out and buy a new body if you break the one you have.

If you want to dance for many years and remain physically active when you stop performing, warming up is essential. Experienced dancers believe that a good warm-up can improve your performance in rehearsals, onstage, and in classes. A good warm-up can also reduce your risk of injury and may extend your performing career (Berardi 2005, 122). Often choreographers cannot take time to warm your body thoroughly. They expect you to be warm and ready to dance when rehearsal begins. As you move into the professional world of dance, it will become your personal and professional responsibility to get your body ready to dance.

Preparing the Body to Move

A good warm-up initiates several changes that prepare the body for movement (Berardi 2005, 123; Fitt 1996, 389–90; White 1996, 129–31). Warm-up increases blood flow to provide the fuel your muscles need to initiate and control movement. Warm-up lubricates your joints so they glide freely and smoothly as you move. Warm-up activates muscles and nerves so they work together to produce coordinated movement. Finally, warm-up focuses your attention on the activity you are about to perform.

Warm-up prepares the body to move:

Increases blood flow (to fuel movement)
Lubricates joints (so they glide freely)
Activates muscles and nerves (that control movement)
Focuses your attention (on the activity you are about to perform)

As you warm up, your body actually *increases in temperature* by a few degrees (Shellock 1983, 134). An indication that your body is getting warm is perspiration, your body's mechanism for cooling itself. As you train, begin to notice which physical activities get you perspiring fairly soon after you begin. Some of these activities may be useful as warm-up exercises. Generally, working the larger muscle groups (such as abdominal and thigh muscles) with control, through a full range of motion, will increase circulation and warm your body quickly. Walking, running, and many conditioning exercises warm the body quickly, as do many large, full-body movement combinations used at the beginning of some technique classes.

Choosing Warm-up Exercises

The principle of specificity (chapter 2) applies to warm-ups as well as to building capacities. The more the warm-up movements mimic the movements you will be performing later (in terms of space, range of motion, tempo, and movement quality), the better they will prepare your body for the stresses of dancing (Franklin 2004, 9). Small, isolated dance movements such as tendue and demi-plié do not move much blood, so they are not sufficient, by themselves, as a warm-up. Include them, but do not rely on them exclusively. To warm your body for dancing, *choose movements that increase blood flow and that feel like dancing.*

Two adjustments to dance movements can increase their usefulness for warm-up. First, the body's relationship to gravity can be changed so the larger muscle groups face a greater than normal challenge. By changing the relationship to gravity, the larger muscles in the torso and thighs are forced to work harder. This may be one reason many dancers like to use floor-barre exercises that incorporate supine, prone, and side-lying positions for warm-up. Second, warm-up *exercises should be slow and controlled to start, and build gradually* to anticipate the type of movements you will be doing while dancing. Ideally, movements like jumping and leaping should not be attempted until the body is quite warm, which may require considerable dancing beyond your initial warm-up. This is probably why such movements come during grande allegro, near the end of ballet classes.

When you have a choice, *moving is better for warm-up* than staying still. This means that holding stretch positions, although generally useful for dancers, should not be your main warm-up activity. You can stretch your muscles by moving slowly and with control through your full range of motion at the hips, spine, shoulders, and feet. Controlled movement will help to warm the muscles as you stretch them. Static stretching (staying in one position for an extended period) will provide greater benefits when your muscles are warm and pliable, so save intensive stretching for your cooldown. If you find yourself saying, "I need to do splits before I am ready to dance," warm up first, then do the splits. Just be careful not to spend all your warm-up time in one or two positions. To warm up, keep moving.

Dancers use a variety of exercises to warm up. Floor-barre, Pilates, and Gyrotonic˚ work (see part 3) are popular among dancers, partly because they have the ability to warm the body thoroughly. Many of our dancers remark that they have their best technique classes after a Pilates, Gyrotonic˚, or Floor-barre workout. They feel more "on their legs" and ready to dance. Several dancer-choreographers, notably Martha Graham and Erick Hawkins, started their technique classes with floor work that offers many of the same benefits. The exercises in the Conditioning Catalog (part 2) are also well suited for warm-up. Try articulated bridging (exercise 3), single and double leg reaches (exercise 5), upper spine extension (exercise 17), and the side legs series (exercise 21) to see whether one of more of these exercises might make a useful addition to your warm-up practice.

As you notice which activities cause your body to perspire, also notice which parts of your body feel ready to move when you finish your warm-up and which parts still feel stiff and unresponsive. Watch other dancers to see what they do. If you have recently changed studios or teachers, notice what is different about what dancers do in your new classes, and consider whether your own warm-up needs to be adjusted to better prepare you for class. If the repertoire is different, your warm-up probably needs to reflect those differences. You may want to ask an experienced dancer to teach you his or her favorite warm-up exercises and include the parts you like best in your own practice.

Design a Personalized Warm-up

If you do not already have your own warm-up, consider building one. You might start by identifying several exercises or movement phrases that involve your whole body and cause you to perspire soon after you begin working. Notice which parts of your body need extra attention to get them ready to dance, and look for movements or exercises that you can add to your warm-up to get those cranky areas prepared to move, too. Once you have collected a bunch of warm-up movements that fit your needs, choreograph them into a continuous sequence you can use to prepare your body to dance. Experiment with sequence, transitions, tempo, and rhythms. If you make your warm-up interesting and continuous, you may be less likely to get distracted partway through and be more likely to be ready to dance when your class or rehearsal begins.

Longer warm-ups, 20 minutes or longer, will get your body better prepared to dance, but they are also more likely to be skipped when time is tight. Make a shorter version so you will have something specific to use when you have less time to warm-up. Emphasize your specific problem areas as well as areas that are likely to be challenged by your current teachers and choreographers.

Start with slow, controlled, full-body movements that emphasize your body's larger muscle groups, pulling against gravity. Save detail work for later in your warm-up and save long-sustained stretches for your cooldown. Rehearse your short warm-up to see if you really can do it in 10

Sample Warm-up

Walk or bicycle to class or rehearsal to get a head start on warming up. Beginning to warm up as you commute means getting multiple benefits from your commute, and it means arriving at the studio closer to being ready to dance.

It will take about 20 minutes to do eight repetitions of each of the exercises below if you work continuously. Use this sample to get ideas for building your own warm-up. If you are not sure exactly what is intended by a specific exercise name, make your best guess, or choose your own exercise to fit your needs.

Starting supine on floor (focus attention and get blood moving using large muscles)

Foot circles and articulation (ex. 2)
Bridging articulated (pelvic curl, ex. 3)
One- and two-leg reaches (ex. 5)
Roll-up with high diagonal reach (ex. 7 and variation)

Sitting cross-legged (activate more muscles that control spine)

Gentle bounce—center, right, left (Hawkins/Graham)
Seated side reaches, add spiraling (Hawkins)
Head swings and circles (ex. 10, variation)

Curled up from supine (challenge torso stabilizing muscles)

Criss-cross (Siler 2000, 70–71)
Hundred (ex. 6) or torso/pelvis stabilization (ex. 14)

Side lying (rehearse disassociation; quiet torso, mobile lower limbs)

Side legs—battement front/back; développé 2nd (ex. 21)

Prone (move spine to end ranges of extension and flexion; refocus attention)

Swan prep (ex. 17)
Kneeling back stretch (ex. 18), eight deep breaths

Pass slowly through . . . on the way to standing (to lengthen hip flexors and hamstrings)

Kneeling hip flexor stretches (ex. 23)
Hamstring stretches (ex. 19)

Standing center (or at barre) (transition to multi-joint, dance-specific movement)

Tendue to plié: parallel—front, side; turned-out—side, back, front
Leg swings—with gentle control throughout
Pliés with relevé suspend—2nd, 1st, parallel
Spine articulation—whole body, moving with control on all three planes of action

or 15 minutes. If you have to rush, identify the most important 10 minutes' worth and use it. When you have plenty of time, do your longer version.

You may want to change your warm-up from season to season, week to week, day to day, or even from teacher to teacher to accommodate the changing demands placed on your body. When you notice special needs in a particular class or rehearsal, adjust your warm-up the following day to accommodate them. Variety will help you stay interested enough to do your warm-up with the integrity needed to guarantee effectiveness.

Transient Effects

Unfortunately, most of the benefits gained from warming up will disappear 15 to 45 minutes after you finish (Clippinger 1988, 77; Shellock 1983, 138). This means that if you perform only in the last half of a long evening program, the company class before the show will be too early to leave your body ready to perform at its peak when you finally get onstage an hour or more later. You will need to rewarm your body before you go onstage. Do you remember how to tell when your body is getting warm?

Cooldown

If you have been dancing hard, your body will recover more quickly and more completely if it is returned to its normal resting state gradually and deliberately (Clippinger-Robertson 1988, 78; Franklin 2004, 11; Wilmore and Costill 2004, 525). An effective cooldown has three general aims: (1) gradually slow blood flow and breathing rate to normal, (2) stretch muscles that were used intensively, and (3) release excess tension acquired while dancing. A cooldown of even a few minutes can help prevent blood from pooling in extremities, which may reduce the amount of soreness you experience later (Fitt 1996, 389; McArdle et al. 2006, 334, 451). Stretching and relaxing can reduce soreness and release tension, rather than allowing it to accumulate.

Cooldown: Three Phases

Gradually return body to pedestrian level of activity
Stretch muscle groups used intensively
Release unnecessary tension

An effective cooldown progresses in the opposite direction of a good warm-up, and it can also be guided by reliance on the principle of specificity. If your class, rehearsal, or performance ends with an especially intense output of energy, start your cooldown by changing gradually from high intensity to the calmness needed for stretching. You might begin by repeating some of the big movements you were just doing and make them progressively slower, calmer, and more elastic with each repetition. The aim is to gradually reduce the size, speed, and intensity of the movements to a level similar to whatever you will be doing next.

As you finish the transition to calmer movement, begin stretching the muscles that were used most intensively while dancing or the muscles that you know normally need to be stretched. Muscle groups that most dancers need to stretch include the hip flexors, hamstrings, calves, hip rotators, lower back, and the front-of-shoulder muscles. Exercises 18 and 23–26 in part 3 cover most of these muscle groups. When cooldown time is limited, recall which muscles have been tight or sore lately, and focus your effort on those muscle groups. Choose some stretches for the muscles that are usually tight or sore on your body and some for those used intensively in the repertory you just performed. Knit the stretches into a seamless sequence,

---

Sample Cooldown

Recovery: 1–2 minutes

Recall a movement phrase (or adagio) done center floor, and repeat a version of it several times, starting at a size, speed, and intensity that nearly matches what you were doing at the end of class, rehearsal, or performance, and changing it gradually to finish with a relatively small, calm, and contained version of the phrase.

Stretches: 3–5 minutes

Hamstring stretch in triangle (ex. 26)—15–30 seconds each leg
Kneeling hip flexor stretch (ex. 23)—15–30 seconds each leg
Splits can count as hamstring and hip flexor stretches on some days
Neck stretches (ex. 10)—15–30 seconds in each of five positions
Arm-over stretch (ex. 24)—15–30 seconds for each arm

Release/relax—2 minutes

Head lift with partner (ex. 30 and chapter 7, table 7.2)
Assist your partner today; receive the favor in return tomorrow
If you are working alone, substitute progressive relaxation (ex. 30, chapter 7, table 7.1)

using the heat your body generated while dancing to help you relax into the stretches. Chapter 7 will offer more suggestions on stretching.

After stretching is an ideal time to rehearse a tension-releasing skill. Taking even a minute to release excess tension can help you reverse the tendency to let it accumulate. If the repertoire you were just performing puts tension in a particular part of the body, do a relaxation exercise. Neck stretches (exercise 10), arm over stretch (exercise 24), or head lift with a partner (see textbox 7.2) might be good choices for releasing tension in the neck and shoulders, for example. If a class or rehearsal creates no special stresses, work on one of the locations where your body normally holds tension. More suggestions will be given in chapter 7.

Some teachers include a cooldown at the end of their technique classes. A former member of the Bella Lewitsky Dance Company once told us that Ms. Lewitsky used to prohibit the audience from coming backstage until her dancers had finished a company cooldown because she believed it helped the dancers recover from the physical stresses of performing. In many situations, dancers have to manage their own cooldown. Some professional dancers credit their cooldown routines with keeping them healthy and extending their dancing careers (Nagrin 1988, 41). Cooling-down after classes, rehearsals, and performances is an investment in your immediate and long-term future.

While it is useful to plan your warm-up, cooldowns are probably best improvised, so you can tailor them to the specific challenges your body faces in class or rehearsal. Use the sensations you feel while stretching and releasing tension to guide you in what to do next. Your body will often tell you, with its response, which activities are most helpful. Cooldown is a good time to trust your intuition.

Making Time

Even the best cooldown routine cannot help if you do not use it. What can you do to make it easier to do a cooldown after classes and rehearsals? Consider listing cooldown in your appointment schedule, working with a partner, keeping a journal or log, or using any other strategies that help you maintain habits that are good for you. If you are tempted to say, "I'm just going to do it this time. I really mean it!" ask whether that approach has worked for you in other situations. If not, think of one small, specific change you can make in how you organize your life that will make your efforts more likely to succeed this time. Once you get in the habit of cooling down after class and feeling the benefits, it will be easier to keep the habit.

Fitting one more thing into a busy dancer's day may seem impossible, but consider the size of the commitment. Assuming 30 seconds per stretch (see chapter 7) times two sides, two to four stretches will take two to four minutes. If you take one or two minutes to gradually calm your body enough to begin stretching and another minute or two to release excess tension, that adds up to just four to eight minutes. If you hear yourself saying, "I don't have time to cool down," consider what you are really saying. Investing a few minutes after dancing to keep your body healthy and performing at its peak may be an opportunity you cannot afford to miss.

References

Berardi, Gigi. 2005. *Finding balance: Fitness and training for a lifetime in dance.* 2nd ed. Pennington, N.Y.: Routledge.

Clippinger-Robertson, Karen. 1988. Principles of dance training. In Priscilla M. Clarkson and Margaret Skrinar, eds., *Science of Dance Training*, 45–90. Champaign, Ill.: Human Kinetics.

Fitt, Sally S. 1996. *Dance kinesiology.* 2nd ed. New York: Schirmer.

Franklin, Eric N. 2004. *Conditioning for dance: Training for peak performance in all dance forms.* Champaign, Ill.: Human Kinetics.

McArdle, William D., Frank I. Katch, and Victor L. Katch. 2006. *Essentials of exercise physiology.* 3rd ed. Baltimore: Lippincott Williams and Wilkins.

Nagrin, Daniel. 1988. *How to dance forever: Surviving against the odds.* New York: Quill.

Shellock, F. G. 1983. Physiological benefits of warm-up. *Physician and Sportsmedicine* 11 (10): 134–39.

White, John. 1996. *Teaching classical ballet.* Gainesville: University Press of Florida.

Wilmore, Jack H., and David L. Costill. 2004. *Physiology of sport and exercise.* 3rd ed. Champaign, Ill.: Human Kinetics.

STUDY GUIDE

1. What are four aims of a well-designed warm-up?

2. What types of exercises work best to get the body warm quickly?

3. Why are the exercises used in the first several minutes of many dance technique classes, such as demi-plié and tendue, not ideal for warming the body quickly?

4. Which is better for warming the body: static stretching or full-body movements performed with control, through a full range of motion? Why?

5. What are the three phases of a well-designed cooldown?

6. What benefits can you expect from cooling down after technique classes, rehearsals, and performances?

7. Outline a 10-minute warm-up to prepare for your hardest class or rehearsal. Rehearse your warm-up to see how long it takes to do it and mark the 10 minutes worth of priority exercises you will do when your warm-up time is limited.

8. List three to five muscle groups that you know would benefit from being stretched after class or rehearsal, and identify a preferred stretch for each muscle group. Complete your cooldown after class or rehearsal and note below any challenges you faced in completing your cooldown.

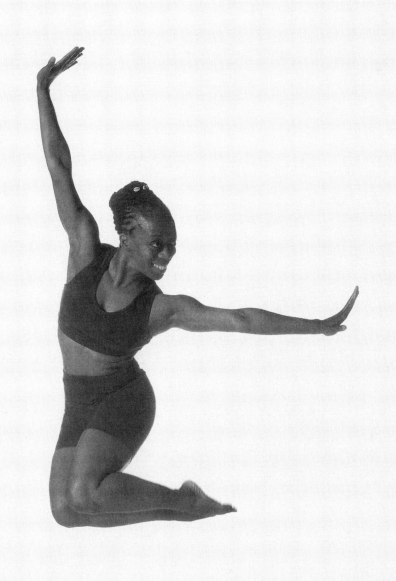

6

Improving Strength and Flexibility

Seven physical capacities dancers must develop and maintain at high levels of performance were described in chapter 1:

Coordination
Alignment
Strength
Flexibility
Endurance
Relaxation
Body composition

This chapter and the next offer suggestions for improving strength, flexibility, endurance, and the ability to release unnecessary tension. Strategies for improving alignment were explained in chapter 4, and help with body composition is given in chapter 8. Training special movement patterns and generally improving neuromuscular coordination will be discussed only briefly in chapter 8 because it is already top priority in most dance technique classes.

Scientific research can provide a foundation from which to create training practices in many physically demanding activities. In comparison with sports, the application of science to the challenges of training dancers is still relatively new, and research results recommending or validating the use of specific dance training approaches are only beginning to appear. Until more research can be conducted with dancers, findings from research with athletes offer some help in determining the best approaches to improving dancer capacities.

It is important to understand, however, that research results are rarely perfectly matched to the training questions we want to answer. Research is conducted under conditions that only approximate the specific circumstances we face when training for dance. So applying research results usually requires interpretation and extrapolation. It is as much art as science. This chapter contains suggestions and guidelines extrapolated from what researchers have learned about training dancers and athletes.[1]

To make them easier to understand, strategies for developing dancer capacities are described separately in these chapters. However, training several capacities simultaneously is often the most efficient way to build them. Employing a holistic approach to training complementary capacities is explained in chapter 7.

Building Strength

Why build strength? This is a topic many dancers, particularly women who are classically trained, try to avoid. They avoid the issue perhaps because strength is associated with masculine features and movement qualities (Andes 1995, 21–24). When we think about strength, we think of the bulky weightlifter who has to turn his whole body to look behind himself. Clearly, that kind of strength is not what dancers need.

Ironically, strength is what makes it possible for dancers to look graceful. Strength allows dancers to lower themselves slowly after relevé without wobbling, without lifting their shoulders, and without making a face. Strength makes it possible for dancers to développé their legs slowly, gracefully, and with unimaginable control to a position where their gesture foot is above their head. Strength also makes it possible to leap to great heights and to land with control. Strength even makes it possible for a dancer to hold a beautifully designed shape so still that a partner can lift him or her effortlessly over head. Of course, the dancer doing the lifting also needs tremendous strength and control to make the lift look effortless. Strength is essential for dance, and the most accomplished dancers are quite strong in special ways.

Strength is also important for avoiding injuries. One likely cause of injuries is asking a muscle to perform an action it is not strong enough to do. Having a little more strength than the minimum needed to get through normal dance movements may reduce injury risk. For example, a dancer with extra strength in the muscles of the lower leg and good proprioception (body position awareness) may be able to pull his foot into neutral alignment to avoid an ankle sprain when he accidentally steps onto a crooked foot. Similarly, dancers who are stronger in the hip flexors that are well positioned to perform the final, highest stage of développé (ilicas and psoas major) may be less likely to develop tendonitis in these and other hip flexors.

Dancers require a highly refined strength. They must strengthen the most efficient muscles for performing each movement to make their movements appear effortless. The most efficient muscles for dance movements are often deep in the body, making them more challenging to recruit than muscles on the surface. Sometimes the best indication that you are working correctly is when a movement seems to happen without any effort. Of course, muscles have to be contracting whenever you move with control, yet some of the most efficient dance muscles are so deep that, when they are strong and their contractions are well coordinated, they do not cause the sensations normally associated with muscular strength.

Improving specific dancer capacities is one purpose for supplemental conditioning. A second purpose is creating general body balance. Both are important.

Using Specificity

Building subtle, refined strength requires attention to detail and the systematic application of conditioning principles. The principle of specificity (explained in chapter 2) is particularly important, and it helps explain some of the limitations for dancers of working in a typical athletic club for building dance-specific capacities. The equipment in commercial gyms is designed to strengthen bodies in safe positions. For example, the squat (plié) machine builds strength in the muscles that extend the ankle, knee, hip, and spine, but it does so in a position that is not well matched to the demands of most concert dance forms. A dancer who stood in squat-machine position during ballet barre would be mistaken for a beginner. Using a squat machine does not develop some of the specific, refined strength needed for plié and other dance movements that use plié. Dancers wanting to strengthen the major extensors of the lower body to facilitate dance movements might be better off doing pliés on a Pilates Reformer, which requires exercisers to hold their bodies in good dancer alignment while the extensor muscles work against spring resistance. Floor-barre exercises and special choreographies by dance training specialists like Irene Dowd can also help dancers develop the refined strength needed for dance.

However, using regular gym equipment can still be helpful to dancers. Dance teacher and exercise physiologist Margaret Wilson points out that dancers who train only in dance positions may exaggerate muscular imbalances that, while specific to dance, can make dancers susceptible to overuse injuries. She believes some amount of training on traditional gym equipment can be healthy for dancers. Taking a similar perspective, PT professor Marjorie Moore told me:

> I agree with Professor Wilson's concern. Dancers overdevelop their quadriceps, hip external rotators [turnout], and ankle plantar flexors [relevé], which become strong within a shortened range of motion.

In addition, many dancers have weakened hamstrings, internal rotators, and ankle dorsiflexors. Both the overly tight and the overly weak
muscles become vulnerable to injuries. Dancers do need to work in
dance-related exercises for part of the day, to develop motor patterns
required for dance; this is a major focus of dance class. Outside of
class, it is important to work the muscles on both sides of the joints,
to rebalance their bodies.

Balancing the two training purposes—doing some work to improve specific dance skills and some work to keep your body balanced—may be the
best overall strategy.

Choosing the right equipment, movement, and alignment are all ways
of using the principle of specificity to guide your dance training. The more
closely your exercises match the demands you will face as a dancer, the
more precisely your conditioning efforts will prepare you to meet those
demands. This is the principle of specificity at work. If you can anticipate
new demands that will be created by new teachers or new repertory, you
can use the principle of specificity to design exercises that will prepare your
body to meet those demands.

Guidelines for Building Strength

1. Use a movement like the dance movement you want to make
   stronger.
2. Use perfect alignment; stop when you can no longer move with
   perfect alignment.
3. Start with a resistance you can move only four times (reps) perfectly.
4. Move with control through the complete range of motion.
5. When four reps are easy, increase to five reps, then six, then
   seven, then eight reps.[2]
6. When eight reps are easy, increase resistance a small amount and
   reduce the reps to four.
7. Keep gradually increasing reps, then resistance until you have a
   little more strength than you think you will need.
8. Train 3 times per week to increase strength.
9. Train 2 times per week to maintain your strength gains.

This general training strategy is based on the principles of conditioning and
is designed to increase strength in ways that are useful to dancers. Steps 1, 2
and 4 are informed by the principle of specificity. To prepare your body for
the demands of dance, you need to do dance-like movements in all the ways

you might be asked to do them while dancing. Alignment has to be close to perfect to be sure you are not rehearsing bad habits. If you cannot maintain good alignment, stop and change the resistance or reduce the number of repetitions; then progress more gradually. Move with control through your complete range of motion to develop and maintain the ability to control movement at any range of motion you might be called on to use.

Applying Adaptation

Steps 3, 7, and 8 are based on the principle of adaptation. Increases in physical capacity, as you remember from chapter 2, result from the body being challenged. Gains are realized largely during the period between workouts, so most muscle groups adapt best when challenged on alternating days (McArdle et al. 2006, 486). If you need to train two days in a row, you can focus on different muscle groups each day to give the muscles you trained yesterday more time to complete their adaptation before you challenge them again tomorrow.

Adding resistance to a movement is the most common approach to increasing challenges when working to build strength. In fact, if you never add resistance, you will limit the level of strength you can develop. Resistance can be increased, to some extent, with creative choreography, as in floor barre and Pilates mat classes. However, external resistance, such as weights, springs and elastic bands, will be needed to optimize strength in many muscle groups.

Choosing the right resistance can be tricky. The objective is to choose a resistance you can move with control and perfect alignment through the complete range of motion only four times. If you choose a resistance you could lift as many as 20 times, for example, you will gain little or no strength from your training efforts because you will not be challenging your body (the principle of adaptation will not be working for you). If you choose a resistance you cannot lift even once without misaligning or holding excessive tension, you will be at risk for teaching your body bad habits and for inviting overuse injuries. Experiment to find a resistance you can almost move perfectly, then go back to the next lower level of resistance and work up to eight perfectly aligned repetitions. When that gets easy, try the next higher resistance again.

Progressing the Overload

Progressive overload (also explained in chapter 2) is the key to consistently and safely improving strength, and it is the guiding principle for steps 5, 6, and 7. Several variables can be changed to adjust overload progressively.

The resistance and the number of reps (repetitions, which is the number of times each movement is repeated) are the most commonly adjusted variables. They should be balanced to offer an overload that is just a little more than your body was able to manage perfectly during your previous workout. If you are worried that you may be increasing too many variables at once and compensating with faulty movement patterns, ask a fitness trainer for help.

Doing four to eight reps will produce complementary gains in strength, muscular endurance, and power if the resistance is set to make one more rep impossible to do perfectly. Once you can do 8 repetitions with a given resistance, increase the resistance by about 5 percent (probably the smallest increment available on the equipment you are using) and reduce the number of repetitions to 4. Pay special attention to alignment, execution, and excess tension, and try to isolate the effort to the part(s) of the body targeted by the exercise. When four reps become easy with the new resistance, increase to five reps, then to six reps and so on. When eight repetitions are easy, increase the resistance another 5 percent and go back to four reps with renewed attention to alignment and perfect execution.

Strength training tradition would suggest doing a second and third set of 4 to 8 repetitions, after a short (30 sec.) rest to permit the body to reset physiologically. Early research showed that doing additional sets lead to more improvement in strength. Recent research is questioning the need for multiple sets (Wilmore and Costill 2004, 107). An alternative is to do a variety of exercises that work the same muscle group. To strengthen the calf muscles, for example, you might do elastic band exercises for the ankles and feet (ex. 11), a relevé-plié exercise on the Pilates Reformer), and one-legged jumps at the barre (variations on ex. 27). Doing three different exercises that work the same group of muscles offers many of the same benefits of doing multiple sets of one exercise, and it has the added advantage of variety, which is good for dancers who may be called on to perform a variety of movements using their calf muscles. The principle of specificity is involved again, but in the opposite direction. Can you figure out how it applies? Try turning the concept of specificity inside out.

Use It or Lose It

The final step in the guidelines for building strength, Step 9, is based on the principle of reversibility, use it or lose it. Once you build strength, you need to continue using it to keep it. Challenging a trained muscle group twice a week is usually enough to maintain its strength. Once a week is better than none at all, but you will probably be losing some capacity in the muscle group if you challenge it only once a week. Think of strength like a bucket with a pin hole in it; you have to keep scooping more in to keep it from running dry.

There are many variations on this general strategy. For example, you will remember that strength is the general term for three related capacities, the other two being muscular endurance and power (can you lift your partner, enough times in a row, and as fast as required by the choreography). The approach described in the guidelines above will produce gains in all three components of strength. However, the principle of specificity can be used to emphasize training for one component or another (e.g., emphasize resistance for strength, repetitions for endurance, and faster movements for power). A fitness trainer can help you decide how to make adjustments to address special needs. If you are unsure, stick with the guidelines to improve strength, muscular endurance, and power. All three components are important for dancers.

If you apply the guidelines consistently, you should begin to notice gains in 5 to 6 weeks, or a little sooner if you are training a muscle group you have never trained before. If you do not seem to be gaining strength or you get a hint of an overuse injury developing (something more than a little soreness or fatigue the day after training) consult a fitness trainer or dance training specialist for help refining your training approach.

Failing in Order to Succeed

In strength training, failure is success (Andes 1995, 26). The most effective way to gain strength is to work the muscle until it cannot work any more, until the point of muscular failure. By pushing the muscles to their limits, the principle of accommodation is invoked, expanding the muscle's capacity to move or resist an outside force. This is how our strength ability grows.

In dance we generally see failure as something to be avoided, and there are some good reasons to avoid failure. For example, when we are onstage, we want to perform the choreography as closely as possible to the choreographer's intent, and when we are in the middle of a double tour en l'air, we want to avoid failing to avoid injury. There are other reasons that we try to avoid failure that may not be so helpful, such as not wanting to risk looking or feeling foolish or trying to maintain an illusion of perfection.

One day when I returned to the beach after a fairly long windsurfing episode, my friend said, "That was great. You didn't fall once." I smiled and said, "I guess that's right," but I had the odd sensation the victory was hollow. I had indeed stayed up the whole trip out but I managed to do so by not taking any real chances, by not stretching my limits, and therefore, not really learning anything new or expanding my abilities. My entire attention was focused on not falling and the tension I felt in my neck and shoulders when I returned to shore reflected that effort.

On my next trip out, I pushed myself to my limits. I sailed on the edge of disaster, trying things I had never done and was not even sure could be done. I fell a lot and returned to shore soaked and smiling. I was exhausted but relaxed and refreshed by the experience. After a long moment, my friend said, "I guess it was tough out there this time." My smile broadened with the satisfaction that I had grown from this windsurfing experience; it would never be the same again.

Learning to tolerate failure in ways that help us grow is an important life lesson. Strength training, particularly when done with a dancer's awareness and demand for ideal alignment and execution, can help us develop this skill, and once developed, we can use it to expand other dance abilities.

Persistent Patience

Once dancers decide a change is needed, they want that change to happen yesterday (Fitt 1996, 369). Of course, the body does not work that way. Your body will gain capacity the quickest and safest when you apply the principles of conditioning by using the guidelines above. Trying to rush a change is a recipe for frustration, the reinforcement of bad habits, and overuse injuries. Consistent effort and persistent patience[3] will allow you to expand your abilities gradually.

Improving Flexibility

Flexibility refers to the capacity to move the various parts of our bodies safely and with control (even when we appear to be out of control) through a full range of motion. It is an ability for which dancers are famous and is exemplified by a développé that places the knee next to the dancer's ear, or an arabesque penché that turns into a vertical split extending from floor to ceiling. Flexibility also allows a dancer to move easily and without restriction through movements that would not look or feel the same in a tighter body.

Experts seem to agree that the healthiest approach to building flexibility is to increase range of motion around a joint, without compromising stability at the joint (Alter 2004, 58; Clippinger 2007, 29; Fitt 1996, 392). A strategy for achieving a healthy balance is to lengthen muscles and their associated connective tissues, and to avoid stretching ligaments. Ligaments hold the ends of bones together, and stretching them can make joints unstable and increase injury risk. *Avoid stretching ligaments and focus instead on lengthening muscle.* Thankfully, ligaments are quite strong and designed to resist stretching. If you use normal stretching exercises and avoid extreme ranges of motion, excessive force, and bad pain, you are not likely to strain ligaments.

Just as bodies adapt to strength demands, they also adapt to the flexibility demands. If you move your joints only through a limited range of motion, the principle of specificity predicts that your muscles will shorten and limit movement to a diminished range of motion (ROM). If you want to have a greater range of motion available to use when you need it, you will have to train your joints to use a greater ROM and continue using that greater ROM to retain the ability to use it. You may ask, "If muscles are too short to permit the use of a larger ROM, how can I train my body to use a greater ROM?" The answer, I hope you have guessed, is progressive overload.[4] Ask your body to move with perfect alignment and execution through a ROM that is just a little greater than what you were able to manage the last time you exercised. Then increase that range of motion, little by little, day by day.

It is generally agreed that ballistic stretching, such as kicking, bouncing, and other fast movement to a joint's range of motion is not the safest way to make a muscle longer. Ballistic movements cause a reflexive contraction of the muscle being stretched, and this response can increase the risk of injuries such as muscle pulls. Some experts believe ballistic stretching contributes to muscle soreness, perhaps due to microscopic tearing of muscle fibers and other connective tissues (Alter 2004, 10; Wilmore and Costill 2004, 99–104). Gentle bouncing, or pulsing, can be useful as warm-up exercise, and ballistic movements are used frequently in dance choreography, so we do not want to avoid using ballistic movements entirely. But they should be rehearsed after your body is quite warm and active, and the more vigorous the movement, the more thorough your warm-up should be before attempting them. Grand battement, for example, comes at the end of barre, and grand jeté usually comes near the end of class. Safer approaches to building flexibility are *slow, sustained stretching* and *proprioceptive neuromuscular facilitation* techniques.

Slow, Sustained Stretching

Slow, sustained stretching (sometimes called passive stretching) involves placing the body in a position that allows gravity to gently pull the targeted muscles longer. A muscle being stretched may contract at first. This reaction is called the stretch reflex. To make muscles longer, it is best to work in cooperation with reflexes. Relaxing into a stretch for 30 to 90 seconds will encourage the release of residual tension in the muscle you are trying to stretch so the muscle can lengthen. Using your breath, especially emphasizing the exhale, can help (Alter 2004, 98–100). It is important to note that relaxing into a stretch involves continual motion, however small. Despite the names given to the techniques below, stretching is not about *holding* a position.

PNF Stretching

PNF stands for proprioceptive neuromuscular facilitation. PNF techniques were developed by physician Herman Kabot in the 1940s and were refined and popularized by physical therapists Margaret Knott, Dorothy Voss, and Margaret Rood. The approach was not designed primarily for stretching, but to address a collection of movement challenges faced by polio, cerebral palsy, and stroke patients (Knott and Voss 1968). Fitness and dance teachers have adapted some of these techniques for use in training athletes and dancers. Although the effectiveness of using these approaches with dancers has yet to be demonstrated empirically, they show enough promise to be included here. If nothing more, they will give you some ideas for how you might expand your own stretching repertoire.

In the first PNF technique, *Hold Relax,* the muscle group you want to stretch is contracted against an immovable resistance (an isometric contraction) for 8 to 10 seconds and then the muscle is relaxed and allowed to lengthen as you move deeper into the stretch. To use this technique to stretch your hamstrings, you might développé one leg toward the ceiling while lying supine and, using your hands to prevent your shin from moving, contract the hamstrings to try to pull the gesture leg away from your face (fig. 6.1a). After 8 seconds of pulling with your hamstrings, and holding with your hands, relax your hamstrings and use your hands to gently pull the same leg toward your face for 30 seconds (fig. 6.1b). If you pull too hard or too fast as you move into the stretch phase, you may activate the stretch reflex and cause a reflexive contraction of the muscles you are trying to lengthen. Think of easing into the stretch and allowing your muscles to get longer. Oppositional pulling concludes with the first phase of this technique; the second phase should relax, as much as possible, the muscle you are trying to stretch (Alter 2004, 158). Everything should be going the same direction. Imagine the hamstrings getting progressively longer to go with the gentle pull of your hands.

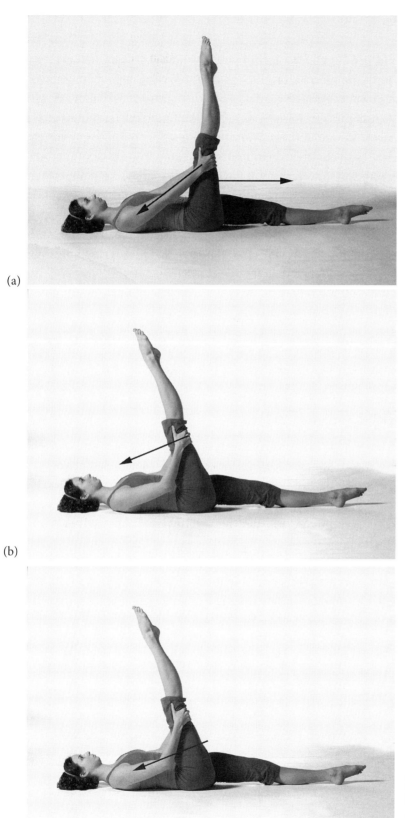

(a)

(b)

(c)

Figure 6.1. PNF stretching: (a) set-up, (b) Hold relax, (c) Slow reversal hold relax.

A second PNF stretching technique, *Slow Reversal Hold Relax,* uses a contraction of the muscles on the opposite side of your body to encourage relaxation of the muscle(s) you are trying to stretch. To stretch the hamstrings using this technique, start by contracting the hamstrings for 8 to 10 seconds, as done in the previous technique (fig. 6.1a), then relax the hamstrings as you contract the muscles on the opposite side of the joint (quadriceps and hip flexors, fig. 6.1c) to deepen the stretch. You might start in the same position but, after pulling with the hamstrings for 8 seconds, relax them and use the muscles at the front of your hip and thigh to pull your shin *toward* your face, deepening the stretch. You can add a gentle pull in the same direction with your hands, but pull only enough to assist the stretch. Keeping your alignment perfectly neutral will intensify the stretch, and it will teach your body to use neutral alignment when working at extreme ranges of motion. This stretch is facilitated by a neurological phenomenon called reciprocal inhibition, in which the muscles on one side of the joint (hamstrings) release when the muscles on the others side (quadriceps or hip flexors) are pulling (McArdle et al. 2006, 394; Moore and Hutton 1980, 322, 26–27).

What Stretching Approach Is Best?

There is debate about which stretching techniques work better for dancers, and it is likely to take some time for researchers to sort this out. You can experiment with your own body to decide which techniques work best for you. You may find that one technique works better in one part of your body while another technique works better in another part of your body. You may find that mixing the techniques helps you lengthen particular muscle groups more effectively than staying with one approach. Most stretching techniques are variations on or combinations of those described above. You may find that just having different ways to stretch on different days helps keep you interested, and that may be the bottom line to stretching effectiveness.

Stretching and Relaxation

Some stretching techniques, particularly those administered by PTs and other manual therapists, are designed to stretch the soft tissue in our bodies, much as we stretch a rubber band. Relaxation of the muscle being stretched is not required to achieve the treatment goal for these techniques. While it has yet to be demonstrated empirically, there appears to be a consensus among experts that relaxation of the target muscles is an important component of self-stretching techniques like those described above. When the target muscle is relaxed, the pull of gravity is safely focused in the belly of the muscle rather than the connective tissue at the end of the muscle (Alter 2004, 158).

If you stay in a hamstring stretch for several seconds, you may feel your hamstrings begin to contract again and your leg may even quiver. The natural tendency at this point is to pull harder, which will probably amplify the stretch reflex and interfere with your stretch. Instead, try releasing the pull of your hands temporarily and relaxing into the stretch again, using a long, slow exhale to release tension in your hamstrings. If the muscles you are trying to stretch seem to relax, keep doing what you are doing. If the muscles you are trying to stretch seem to be getting tenser, come out of the stretch, relax a few seconds, and restart the stretch. Dance exercise physiologist, Karen Clippinger (2007, 67) recommends repeating each stretch twice, for 30 seconds, with a brief rest between. Another approach is to repeat the cycle of relaxing and restarting until you have stretched the targeted muscle for 30 to 90 seconds in all. Classical ballet teacher John White (1996, 135) recommends holding a position that stretches a muscle 80 percent, 90 percent, and then 100 percent of it normal maximum length for 3 to 5 seconds, relaxing briefly between repetitions. He suggests repeating the pattern with holds of 8 to 10 seconds and aiming for the final stretch to be slightly beyond the muscle's normal range of motion.

In the release portion of the stretches described above, your aim is to relax the muscle you are trying to stretch while allowing gravity to help lengthen it. Stretching is usually considered passive and indirect, but it is also active, in the sense that you have to continually search for ways to allow your muscles to relax and lengthen. This Zen-like aspect can make stretching difficult for dancers who are overly concerned with being in control and those who are easily distracted. To make the most of your stretching time, keep noticing whether you are relaxing into the stretch, and resist the temptation to force your body into a more extreme range of motion if it seems to increase tension in the muscles you are trying to lengthen. Stretching is a dynamic, interactive process. Think of it as a dialog with your own body.

In her textbook *Dance Kinesiology,* Sally Fitt suggests "nudging around" when stretching. What she means is adjusting your position slightly and repeatedly until you find a position that lengthens the target muscle(s), staying there for several seconds, and then adjusting some more. Using this approach, you may have a slightly different position every day, or even a continuously changing position during a single stretch. You will be refining the stretch to fit your body and the way it feels *at that moment*. This activity will help you develop heightened sensitivity to how your body feels from moment to moment, which is a useful skill in its own right.

Other fitness specialists recommend breathing into a stretch, reaching or moving through a stretch, and noticing how the sensations change from moment to moment (Alter 2004, 151; Franklin 2004, 81–82; Hackney 1998, 53). All are strategies for encouraging the release of muscular tension so the targeted muscles can lengthen. Experiment with various approaches to evolve a personal strategy that works for you. When you are having a tense day and your old strategies do not seem to be working, go back to experimenting. The goal is to release tension so you can relax into a stretch. Use the sensations in your own body as your guide.

Good Pain/Bad Pain

Good and bad pain were discussed in chapter 3, and it was suggested they be used to guide your training efforts as you return from injury. Good and bad pain can also be used to guide your strength-building and flexibility-enhancing efforts. The mild *burning* sensation that occurs in the whole muscle when doing strengthening exercises, or the *tingling* sensation that occurs across the belly of a muscle when it is being stretched, are indicators that you are helping your body adapt to new challenges. Sharp pain, focused close to the joint and occurring when working with too great a resistance or forcing your body into too extreme a position, is a signal to change the way you are working. Adjust your position or the amount of resistance until the sharp pain is replaced with one of the *good pain* sensations. Use good pain to guide your strengthening and stretching efforts (Fitt 1996, 370).

How Often and When to Stretch

Stretching twice a day is a reasonable approach for most dancers who are trying to increase range of motion. Stretching too often can irritate muscles and tendons by robbing them of the rest they need to recover during and between classes, rehearsals and workouts. Stretching less often may be sufficient for dancers who are just trying to keep an already sufficient range of motion. Every body's response to stretching is unique, so notice and keep doing what works for you.

When to stretch is an important question for dancers. Muscles stretch best when they are warm, like right after a technique class, rehearsal, or conditioning workout (White 1996, 135). The heat generated by exercise makes muscles more pliable and more willing to stretch. Don't waste the heat it took you an hour or more to build in class. Invest it in making your tightest muscles a little longer and more relaxed. Only half kidding, Michael Alter suggests you stretch "whenever you feel like it" (2004, 154). For dancers who are *flexibility challenged*, this may be the best advice of all.

There is some evidence that intensive stretching can compromise performance that involves muscular power (remember strength, muscular endurance, and power) (Alter 2004, 156; Deighan 2005, 16). If stretching just before the parts of class that require strong, fast movements such as jumping, seem to compromise your performance, try doing some controlled movement through a full range of motion as preparation and save intensive stretching for after the power activity.

Dance PT Craig Phillips told me that there is some concern that especially long or intense stretching might irritate nerves and cause muscles being stretched to contract to protect themselves. Ironically, dancers who are normally quite flexible may be more susceptible to this problem. If you are stretching long and hard and seem to be getting tighter rather than more flexible, try reducing how hard and long you stretch to see if that helps. If it does not, consult a physical therapist or fitness trainer to get help in refining your stretching approach.

Passive and Active Range of Motion

Achieving the extreme ranges of motion used in dance choreography requires length in the muscles on one side of a joint and strength in the muscle on the other side. If a dancer can lift her leg to a high second position with her foot above her shoulder using her hand, but can only lift her leg to a little above waist level without help from her hand, she has greater passive than active range of motion (Clippinger-Robertson 1986). This dancer might do well to spend a little more time strengthening the muscles that lift the leg, even if that requires cutting back modestly on stretching time.

Guidelines for Improving Flexibility

1. Determine which muscles need to be lengthened.
2. Focus stretch on muscles, rather than joints and ligaments.
3. Warm your muscles by taking class, working out, or doing your own warm-up.
4. Find a position that allows gravity to gently pull the targeted muscles longer.
5. Relax into the stretch, allowing it to deepen as tension subsides.
6. Use a PNF techniques to facilitate the stretch.
7. Make adjustments that encourage the release of tension.
8. Continue the stretch for 30 to 90 seconds.

9. Stretch again today, if you need to increase your flexibility.

10. Stretch every day, especially if flexibility is hard for you to maintain.

Seeking Balance

Increasing flexibility without limits may predispose dancers to injuries (Deighan 2005, 14). Instead, the goal should be to acquire enough Range of motion to execute dance movement without undue restriction. Striking a balance is the goal. Likewise, developing the strength needed to control movement in an expanded range of motion, may be key to minimizing injury risks (Alter 2004, 166). Building strength and flexibility were discussed together in this chapter to emphasize their mutually supportive relationship. Interaction in the development of the capacities will be discussed in the next chapter.

Notes

1. The recommendations for building strength and flexibility were clarified and enhanced with suggestions from Margaret Wilson, associate professor of theater and dance at the University of Wyoming in Laramie, and Marjorie Moore, associate professor of physical therapy at St. Catherine College in Minneapolis.

2. I stop at eight repetitions because many dancers lose concentration when a simple movement is repeated too many times. It may be that a low tolerance for repetition is one reason dancers become dancers instead of distance runners or swimmers. PTs and fitness trainers often increase repetitions to 15 or 20 per set and total repetitions to as many as 50 to encourage the development of muscular endurance. If you can stay focused and maintain ideal alignment, feel free to work beyond eight reps.

3. I was introduced to the concept of persistent patience by Jack McLanahan, who devoted his career to creating credit unions for low-income citizens in central Kentucky.

4. Alter (2004, 145) suggests using the term *over-stretching* to refer to the load or challenge that is adjusted during flexibility training. The concept is the same.

References

Alter, Michael J. 2004. *The science of flexibility*. 3rd ed. Champaign, Ill.: Human Kinetics.
Andes, Karen. 1995. *A woman's book of strength*. New York: Berkley.

Clippinger, Karen. 2007. *Dance anatomy and kinesiology.* Champaign, Ill.: Human Kinetics.

Clippinger-Robertson, Karen. 1986. Increasing functional range of motion in dance. *Kinesiology and Medicine for Dance* 8 (3): 8–10.

Deighan, Martine A. 2005. Flexibility in dance. *Journal of Dance Medicine & Science* 9 (1): 13–17.

Fitt, Sally S. 1996. *Dance kinesiology.* 2nd ed. New York: Schirmer.

Franklin, Eric N. 2004. *Conditioning for dance: Training for peak performance in all dance forms.* Champaign, Ill.: Human Kinetics.

Hackney, Peggy. 1998. *Making connections: Total body integration through Bartenieff fundamentals.* Amsterdam: Gordon and Breach.

Knott, Margaret, and Dorothy E. Voss. 1968. *Proprioceptive neuromuscular facilitation: Patterns and techniques.* 2nd ed. New York: Harper and Row.

McArdle, William D., Frank I. Katch, and Victor L. Katch. 2006. *Essentials of exercise physiology.* 3rd ed. Baltimore: Lippincott Williams and Wilkins.

Moore, Marjorie A., and Roger S. Hutton. 1980. Electromyographic investigation of muscle stretching techniques. *Medicine & Science in Sport & Exercise* 12 (5): 322–29.

White, John. 1996. *Teaching classical ballet.* Gainesville: University Press of Florida.

Wilmore, Jack H., and David L. Costill. 2004. *Physiology of sport and exercise.* 3rd ed. Champaign, Ill.: Human Kinetics.

STUDY GUIDE

1. Why do many dancers avoid the topic of building strength?

2. How can building strength benefit dancers?

3. What are some differences between the type of strength dancers need and the type of strength other athletes need?

4. Summarize the guidelines for building strength in three or four sentences.

5. Explain how one of the principles of conditioning applies to one of the guidelines for building strength.

6. What is one good way for dancers to do multi-set exercises?

7. About how long does it take to achieve a noticeable change in strength, and what are the risks of trying to rush it?

8. Which body tissues should be targeted for safe stretching? Which body tissue should dancers specifically avoid stretching?

9. Briefly describe three stretching methods that are preferred over ballistic stretching.

10. When will working on flexibility have the most benefit for dancers?

11. Summarize the guidelines for stretching in two or three sentences.

12. Why would doing different exercises to work the same muscle group be useful to dancers? How does the principle of specificity help explain why this is true?

7

Improving Endurance and Releasing Tension

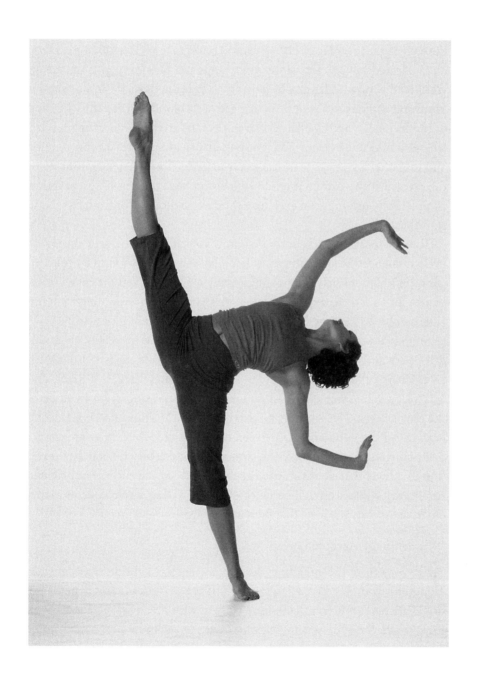

This chapter offers guidance for developing aerobic endurance and releasing unnecessary tension. It also explains why training complementary capacities may be the most effective way to make changes, and it offers suggestions for avoiding overtraining by training in cycles.

Improving Aerobic Endurance

Aerobic capacity is sometimes called cardiorespiratory endurance or cardiovascular endurance. It is your body's ability to supply your muscles with the oxygen they need to continue working over extended periods. This ability is affected by how efficiently your lungs can take oxygen from the air you breathe, how well your blood can absorb the oxygen, how well your heart and arteries can pump the oxygen-rich blood to your muscles, and how effectively your capillaries can release the oxygen into your muscles. It is also affected by how efficiently your blood absorbs carbon dioxide and the other by-projects of muscular activity, how efficiently your veins can transport the carbon dioxide-rich blood back to your lungs, and how completely your lungs can exchange the carbon dioxide for fresh oxygen to start the cycle over.

The efficiency of each body system involved in the oxygen-supplying cycle influences aerobic fitness. When challenged by working a little longer or more intensively than you normally work, your aerobic capacity expands. Of course, if you stop challenging your cardiorespiratory systems, your aerobic capacity will diminish (in other words, use it or lose it).

Studies have found that dancers, as a group, are not especially fit aerobically, perhaps because the work in most technique classes is not designed to challenge the cardiorespiratory systems (Cohen, Segal, Witriol, and McArdle 1982; Wyon 2005). Although dancers do work intensely in class, the intensity usually lasts only a short time (16–32 jumps or a 15–20 second grand allegro combination). Between exercises and while other groups are performing a center or traveling combination, dancers reduce their exertion to a level that does not use much oxygen, so the cardiovascular and respiratory systems are not being challenged. To train these systems, dancers have to work at a level that demands energy for an extended period.

Why Train the Aerobic Energy Systems?

Before looking at the guidelines for training aerobic capacity, let's consider a question you may be asking yourself. If the aerobic energy systems are not challenged much in technique classes, why do dancers need to train them at all? There are several reasons. First, as you know, performing some dances requires a more aerobic effort than is common in technique classes. To improve the ability to perform aerobically demanding choreography, dancers must train their aerobic systems. Second, aerobically fit dancers are able to continue working at high effort levels over longer periods, such as evening-long performances and all-day residency rehearsals (Wyon 2005, 8–9). In addition, dancers who are not aerobically fit get fatigued sooner and, at the end of long performances and rehearsals, are more likely to compromise their alignment and the execution of movements that they can perform perfectly when they are fresh. This pattern invites injuries. Finally, aerobic training is key to maintaining healthy body composition.

Improving Aerobic Capacity

The general recipe for improving aerobic capacity is to engage in an activity that increases your heart rate to about 75 percent of its maximum level and to sustain that level of activity for 20 to 30 minutes three or more times per week. You might start with an activity that uses the larger muscles of the body in some rhythmic motion. Jogging, bicycling, and swimming are probably the most common aerobic training activities because they use the body's larger muscle groups, and the movements can be repeated continuously for long periods. Walking also trains aerobic capacity, especially if you walk long enough, fast enough, or go uphill. There is a vast array of other aerobic training activities, including aerobic dance, rowing, and cross-country skiing, and there are many variations on the main themes of jogging and biking such as stair stepping, spinning, treadmill work, and elliptical training. Games that employ repetitive movements using larger muscle groups such as basketball, tennis, soccer, and water polo can also have an aerobic training effect if done continuously for 20 minutes or more, at a level that causes your heart to work in the aerobic training range. British professors Matt Wyon and Emma Redding and their colleagues at the Laban Center in London and the University of Wolverhampton north of London have been working to develop aerobic training movement combinations that can be incorporated into modern dance classes to achieve a training effect that is well matched to the demands of dance (Wyon, Redding, Abt, Head, and Sharp 2003).

Exercise Duration

Efficiency advocates have detected aerobic training effects with workouts as short as 15 minutes of continuous exercise. Certainly, it is better to do a short workout than none at all, but to get the level of benefit dancers need will require an investment of a little more aerobic training time.

At the other extreme, some endurance athletes (runners, cyclists, triathletes) train many hours each day. Such a training approach would yield greater aerobic training benefits, but the time required to do it would compete with other demands on dancers' time. Striking a balance is again the best guiding principle. Dancers need enough aerobic activity to build their aerobic endurance to a level a little greater than what they will need while rehearsing or performing, but they cannot train so much that they compromise their dance training or increase their risk of injury.

The general guideline of 20–30 minutes of aerobic activity offers a reasonable balance for dancers, although those who have not engaged in aerobic training recently will want to work up to this level gradually over a period of six weeks or more (Koutedakis et al. 1999; Wyon 2005). If you find this duration is not quite enough, like when you know you will have to perform a 45-minute aerobically demanding dance later in the season, or when you will be participating in a weeklong residency with a guest artist who will be setting an aerobically demanding work, increase the length of your aerobic workouts gradually until you reach a level sufficient to give you a little more capacity than you think you will need. Having a little extra capacity to draw on in unusual circumstances is good insurance.

Exercise Frequency

A workout frequency of three times per week is the typical recommendation for promoting adaptation of the C-R (cardiorespiratory) system (McArdle et al. 2006, 448). Exercising five times a week may produce faster improvement, but that many aerobic workouts may begin to compete with your dance training and increase your chances of developing overuse symptoms. Consider using times when you are on a break from normal dancing (holidays, summers, off-season) to increase your aerobic training to four or five times a week to accelerate progress. Then return to three aerobic workouts a week during your dancing season. Working once or twice a week will probably not increase your aerobic capacity, but it may help you keep the level of aerobic fitness you already have or slow its deterioration (remember the leaky bucket analogy from the chapter 6). Some exercise is better than none, especially if you expect to return to more frequent workouts when your professional life permits you to do so. If you get stuck at one aerobic workout a week for several months, you may want to work with a fitness trainer to refine your overall training approach.

Making It Work

Probably the most important factor in succeeding at aerobic training is selecting a training activity you can tolerate doing for 20–30 minutes at a time. With the diversity of aerobic training equipment available in gyms these days, the variety of teachers leading fitness classes, and the collection of independent fitness activities available to choose from, there should be a number of aerobic activities any dancer can tolerate, and maybe even enjoy, for 20-30 minutes at a time. Jogging or hiking outdoors, for example, may offer a good balance to the intensive indoor studio work dancers face on a daily basis. You can even piece together a variety of activities for your aerobic training program to stay interested across weeks or even during a single workout (e.g., bike for 10 minutes, row for 5 minutes, and walk for 5 more minutes). One caution is to incorporate each new activity gradually so your body has time to adapt to the new stresses it will be learning to manage. This is as important when changing aerobic activities as it is when changing dance styles, choreographers, or technique teachers.

Adjusting your level of effort while training is another key to success in aerobic training. A target of 75 percent of your maximum heart rate is ideal, but aerobic training effects can be achieved with effort levels from 55 percent to more than 90 percent of maximum heart rate. The principle of specificity (see chapter 2) can help you select a target training range that is matched to your current abilities and to your ultimate goals. Working at higher heart rates is not necessarily better. Higher levels use more oxygen and burn more calories per minute, but the activity cannot be sustained as long. Working at lower levels uses less oxygen and burns fewer calories per minute, but it also allows our bodies to use more fat as fuel, a connection that will be addressed in chapter 8. Gradually build up to 20 minutes of continuous exercise at 75 percent of your maximum heart rate, three days per week, then consult a fitness trainer to get help in fine-tuning your program to match your specific needs.

The need to build aerobic training programs gradually (using the progressive overload principle, explained in chapter 2) cannot be overemphasized. Starting too ambitiously can invite overuse injuries and encourage quitting (McArdle et al. 2006, 438, 450; Pollock 1988, 271–72). Working at 60 percent of your maximum heart rate, 5–10 minutes each workout, two or three times during your first week should be plenty if you have not engaged in aerobic training recently. From there, you can increase your training workload a small amount each week, until you reach your training target. It is important to note that effort level (intensity), duration, and number of workouts per week all contribute to your total workload. Their combined effect is what must be increased gradually. If you notice any overuse symptoms, such as inflammation or accumulating soreness, reduce your workload and progress more gradually. If you need help adjusting your workload, ask a fitness trainer for help. This is the type of assistance they are trained to provide.

Heart Rate

If you are going to exercise at a level that causes your heart to pump at 75 percent of your maximum heart rate, you need to know how to estimate your maximum heart rate. Hearts are pumps that run faster when our bodies demand more energy for muscular contraction and movement. As we work harder, our hearts pump faster. However, our hearts have a maximum speed that is governed largely by age. Your maximum heart rate can be measured directly by lab or clinic technicians who will put you on a treadmill or stationary bicycle (called an ergometer, literally "work-meter," in exercise physiology labs) where the workload can be increased gradually as your heart rate is monitored using an electrocardiograph (ECG). As the workload increases, your heart rate will increase correspondingly until it reaches a plateau. If the workload is increased further after your heart reaches its maximum rate, your muscles will not be able to get the fuel they need to continue operating at such a high level. Since your heart is a muscle, too, your heart rate may even decrease when it reaches maximum, and you will probably decide to quit working because it doesn't feel good. If you are wearing a gas exchange analyzer, the technicians can calculate the amount of oxygen your body is able to process as your heart rate peaks. This is called volume of maximal oxygen uptake (VO_2max), and it is generally considered the most valid measure of aerobic fitness (Wilmore and Costill 2004, 290).

You can see that measuring maximum heart rate directly is an involved process. While it would be interesting to do it at some point, it is not something you will want to do regularly. A practical alternative is to estimate maximum heart rate (MHR). The simplest formula for estimating is

$$220 - (\text{your age}) = \text{estimated MHR}$$

in beats per minute (bpm). The formula for determining your *aerobic training target* is:

$$\text{MHR} \times 75 \text{ percent} = \text{Aerobic Training Target}$$

These two formulas can be combined into one:

$$(220 - \text{Age}) \times .75 = \text{Aerobic Training Target}$$

There are other, more involved approaches to determine an aerobic training target, but this one will get you close enough to begin training. Remember that if you have not been engaging in aerobic training recently, you will need to begin at a lower intensity, 55–60 percent of MHR, and work up to 75 percent over several weeks. An example may clarify how this formula can be used to determine a dancer's aerobic training target. Suppose we have a 20-year-old dancer who wants to increase her aerobic capacity. The calculation would go like this:

$$(220 - 20) \times .75 = 150 \text{ bpm} = \text{Aerobic Training Target}$$
$$(220 - 20) \times .60 = 120 \text{ bpm} = \text{Initial Training Level}$$

Building Aerobic Capacity

To build a base level of aerobic fitness, this 20-year-old dancer might begin exercising for 5 to 10 minutes at a level that causes her heart to work at 120 beats per minute, and repeat that workout two more times the first week. She might increase her workout time by a few minutes the second week and, if all goes well, increase her workout duration a few minutes more the third and subsequent weeks until she reaches 20–30 minutes. Then she might pick up the pace just a little to cause her heart to work at 125 or 130 beats per minute during at least part of her workout. She could continue to gradually increase her pace, aiming to reach her 75 percent aerobic training target of 150 beats per minute 6 to 10 weeks after starting training.

Many of the aerobic training machines in fitness centers have heart rate monitors built into their consoles. Sensors are sometimes imbedded in handle bars that you hold for 8 to 10 seconds while the machine measures your pulse in beats per minute. Your pulse is displayed on the machine's console with other workout statistics. There are also portable heart rate monitors that can be strapped around the bottom of the rib cage. They either connect to a wrist watch that displays your pulse or can transmit their measurements directly to the console on the exercise machine.

While electronic pulse monitors are convenient and fun to use occasionally, there are less involved techniques for measuring heart rate. One simple approach is to slow down or pause briefly and take your pulse for 6 seconds. *Adding a zero to the number of beats you count in 6 seconds will give you a quick estimate of your heart rate in beats per minute.* This type of measurement is not as precise as an electronic monitor, but it is close enough to let you know whether you need to work a little harder or back off some. As you gain experience with aerobic training and the specific exercises you have chosen to use, you will learn to sense when you are working at just the right level of intensity. Then you can just check your guesses with one of the methods above periodically to calibrate your senses. So do not delay starting your aerobic training program while you wait for Santa to bring you a new heart rate monitor.

How Hard to Work

A common mistake in beginning an aerobic training program is working too hard (Pollock, 1988, 266, 268). A good rule of thumb is that you should feel you are working hard, but you should be able to carry on a conversation with a training partner (McArdle et al. 2006, 448). If you cannot talk, you are probably working too hard; slow down and enjoy the activity and your partner's company. Remember that your body is a physiological system, and it will improve its capacities fastest and safest when you gradually increase the challenge you ask it to manage.

Guidelines for Increasing Aerobic Capacity

1. Select an aerobic activity you can tolerate for 20–30 minutes at a time.
2. Calculate your MHR and your aerobic training target (75 percent of MHR).
3. Purchase or borrow protective equipment (e.g., good shoes for running).
4. Warm up before you begin exercising.
5. Start with a short workout (5–10 minutes) at a mildly elevated heart rate (55–60 percent of MHR).
6. Gradually increase frequency, duration, and intensity of workouts, one variable at a time.
7. Build to 20–30 minutes at 75 percent of MHR over a period six weeks or more.
8. Exercise two or three times a week during your dancing season; four or five times a week during off-season.
9. If overuse symptoms appear, reduce your workload and progress more gradually.
10. After 10–12 weeks, have a fitness trainer help you refine your program.

Refining your C-R Training Approach

When you are pushing your body especially hard (petite and grand allegro work such as jetés and lifts, for instance), some of the energy your muscles need to move your body comes from fuel that is stored in the muscle fibers and blood cells. This type of fuel does not need oxygen to produce energy, so it is called anaerobic (i.e., without oxygen). Anaerobic energy systems can provide bursts of energy for intense movement, but that energy lasts only for short periods (up to about 10 seconds). Your anaerobic energy systems get trained to some degree whenever you are physically active, and as the principle of specificity would dictate, your anaerobic abilities will adapt to match the type of activity you engage in regularly.

At the beginning of the chapter, it was mentioned that a lot of dance activity is episodic. You work hard for a while, making greater use of your anaerobic energy systems, and then you work easier for a while, relying primarily on your aerobic energy systems. Once you have established a sound foundation of aerobic fitness, you may want to refine your C-R program to include training that mimics the type of performing you do. A fitness trainer can help you create an interval training program to help your body get the most out of all its energy systems (McArdle et al. 2006, 456; Wilmore and Costill 2004, 196; Wyon 2005).

Releasing Unnecessary Tension

The ability to release unnecessary tension is a skill many dancers can benefit from improving. Releasing excess tension can have the simple therapeutic effect of reducing discomfort (e.g., in the neck and shoulders). It is also key to moving efficiently, which can make training, rehearsing, and performing less effortful and leave your muscles fresh and ready to work at their best when needed. Moving efficiently can reduce stresses that shorten muscles and make them tense. Being able to move with less tension can allow dancers to perform movement qualities that tense bodies cannot achieve. Finally, letting go of unnecessary tension can help dancers look and feel calm, composed, and confident—ready to meet the next challenge that comes their way.

Getting Started

Like other physical capacities, the ability to release unnecessary tension can be improved with practice. Full body relaxation is a good way to begin to learn tension releasing techniques. The difference between holding tension and releasing it may be easier to detect when the whole body is involved.

More than 70 years ago, University of Chicago researcher Edmund Jacobsen began developing full body relaxation techniques (Jacobson 1938). One of his techniques, progressive relaxation, involves actively increasing tension in an isolated body part, holding it for several seconds, and then releasing the tension. The doer is able to experience the difference in the body part while consciously tensing and then relaxing it. The doer can also compare the sensation in the tensed part with the parts of the body that have already been relaxed and the parts that have yet to be relaxed. Part by part, the body as a whole becomes progressively more relaxed.

The experience of being led through a relaxation session of this type is luxurious. Having a teacher or trainer lead you will probably feel the best because you will be free to pay attention to how your body is reacting, instead of thinking about what comes next. If you do not have a teacher to lead you, you may want to purchase a commercially produced audio recording (see Resources, part 3) to serve as your guide, or you might ask your teacher if you may record a class relaxation session so you can use the recording to practice your tension releasing skills at home. You might even make your own audio recording to use to talk yourself into relaxing. To get the timing and tone right, make your recording while leading a friend or relative through a relaxation session. An outline for a progressive relaxation session is provided in the text box below.

Progressive Relaxation

Instructions

Unless you are in a very warm room, put on some socks or slippers, long pants or leg warmers, and a long-sleeved shirt to keep your body from becoming chilled. Relaxation can reduce blood flow to the extremities, causing you to feel chilled, even if you feel warm when you begin.

Start with this script and allow your words to adapt and change to match your personal preferences. Try using the script to help a friend relax and record it so you can play it back to help yourself relax later. When you play it back, imagine that someone else is giving the instructions. Instead of critiquing your reading performance, focus on following the instructions and tuning in to the sensations they create.

It's important not to rush a relaxation session. To establish a good pace, watch those you are leading and move on when you feel they are ready to go with you. This whole outline should take 20 minutes or perhaps a little longer the first time you do it. If you don't have time to do it all, choose a focus: lower body, upper body, or torso, neck, and head. Save the full outline for a day when you have enough time to do it leisurely. It is easier to relax when you do not feel rushed.

Script

Begin lying supine on a mat, arms by your sides, palms facing the ceiling, and eyes closed. If you can extend your hips and knees without causing pain in your lower back, do so. Otherwise, use constructive rest position (exercise 1 in part 2). Focus on your breathing to start, allowing it to deepen and extending the exhalation. Notice how your breathing moves your ribs and spine. Try to let go of any tension you notice, but do not worry if it does not release immediately.

Focus on your left hand and make it into a fist. Grip it tighter . . . tighter . . and still tighter (4–6 seconds altogether). Then let the tension go and let your fingers unfold like the petals of a flower opening to meet the sun. Take a deep breath in . . . and a breath out, letting go of any tension in your left hand.

Press the back of your left wrist into the mat and tense the muscles in your forearm, upper arm, and shoulder, making them more tense . . . even more tense . . . tenser still (4–6 sec) . . . and let the tension go with a deep breath in . . . and out. Take another deep breath in . . . and out.

[Repeat with right hand, then with the arm.]

Grip the toes on your right foot to make it feel like a fist. Grip it tighter . . . and tighter . . . and still tighter . . . then release it. Take a deep breath in . . . and as you exhale, let go of any tension in your right foot.

Press your right heel into the floor and pull your toes toward your knee, creating tension in lower leg. Make it tighter . . . and tighter . . . even tighter . . . then release it. Take a deep breath in . . . and out, letting go of any tension from your knee down.

Tense the muscles in your right thigh—the front . . . back . . . inside and outside. Make your whole right thigh tenser . . . and tenser . . . and tenser . . . and release it. Take a deep breath in . . . and out.

[Repeat with left foot, lower leg, and thigh.]

Grip the muscles on the back of your pelvis (your gluteals). Squeeze them tight . . . tighter . . . tightest . . . then release them and take a deep breath in . . . and out.

Scoop out your belly, pulling your lower back toward the mat. Imagine your belly button is tied to a string that someone is pulling from below the floor. Tense all the muscles in your abdominal wall, making them tighter . . . tighter . . . still tighter . . . and release them with a deep breath in . . . and an extended breath out.

Squeeze the shoulder blades (scapulae) together, and imagine your breast bone (sternum) is attached to a hook extending from the ceiling that is lifting only your chest. Make the muscle around your rib cage—the back, front, left side, and right side—tense . . . tenser . . . even tenser . . . and release, using the breath out to let go of any tension in this part of your body.

Press the back of your head gently into the mat and roll it slowly from side to side, increasing the pressure gradually and making the muscles in the back of your neck tenser . . . and tenser . . . and still tenser . . . and let them go.

Bring your chin toward your chest, tensing the muscles on the front of your neck, making them tense . . . more tense . . . more tense . . . and, if your head is off the floor, let it float gently back to the mat and release any tension in your neck as you breathe deeply in . . . and out.

Open your mouth as wide as you can, open your eyes as wide as you can, stick out your tongue as far as you can, and tense every muscle in your face. Imagine you are roaring like a lion . . . then release the tension and let your eyes close. Continue breathing deeply, letting any remaining tension dissolve with each breath out (3–5 breath cycles).

Let's inventory the various parts of your body to notice and release any remaining tension. Do not feel you have to move the body part to show that you are letting tension go. Your private experience is what counts. Just feel the release.

Start with the right foot, lower leg, knee, thigh, and hip—the whole right leg. If there is any tension in that part of your body, just let it go.

[Repeat for the left side.]

Let the muscles on the back of your pelvis soften and spread wide on the floor. No one is looking, so take this opportunity to let them relax.

Check your belly and lower back. If there is any tension in this part of your body, let it go.

Check the muscles around your rib cage . . . the front, back, right side, and left side. If there is any tension around your rib cage, just let it go.

Now your neck—front back, both sides. If there is any tension there, let it go.

Left hand, wrist, forearm, upper arm, and shoulder. . . . If there is any tension, let it go.

[Repeat for right hand, wrist, upper arm, and shoulder.]

Finally check your head and face and let go of any tension you find there. Feel wide across your forehead, and let your eyebrows drift down as if to cover your eyes. Let your cheeks droop down toward the floor. Allow your jaw to drop and your teeth and lips to separate slightly. Let your tongue drop back into your mouth.

Continue to breathe deeply in . . . and out . . . letting go of any remaining tension in your body. Appreciate the sensation as you continue to breathe deeply.

[Stay at this phase 3–5 minutes before proceeding. Increase duration gradually across episodes or adjust to match time available on each occasion.]

Progressive Relaxation continued

> Listen to the next set of instructions and follow them at a pace that feels leisurely to you; do not rush. To go on with your day, you will need to put a little tension back into your body. Start by slowly wiggling a finger or toe. Let the movement in this isolated part of your body get bigger and begin to cause other parts of your body to move. Continue until your whole body is gently writhing as it might when awakening from a nap on a lazy afternoon. Trust your body to move in ways that are good for it, and notice how your body wants to move as it returns from deep relaxation.
>
> Once your body has stretched in several directions, allow it to come to rest, lying in a curled position on one side. Take your time to come to sitting, then kneeling, and finally standing. Work at your own pace; there is no need to rush. If you can afford to stay relaxed, take the sensation with you into your next activity. If you have to be at full attention, *march* around the room for a minute or two at 80 steps per minute (march tempo) to bring your tension closer to your normal level.

Isolated Relaxation

Learning to relax isolated body parts, particularly those that readily retain excess tension such as the neck, shoulders, lower back, and hips, is another relaxation skill useful to dancers. In addition to making movement more efficient, learning to release isolated tension can help you use that ability while dancing to achieve qualities of movement that are not possible when too much tension is present.

An isolated relaxation approach that works well for dancers is the *lifts*, a series of partnered exercises described by Sally Fitt (1996, 130–36) and based on the work of Moshe Feldenkrais (1977). The lifts encourage the release of tension in isolated body parts by giving a helper responsibility for holding and gently moving your head, leg, or scapula (shoulder blade). Your assignment, as the dancer being lifted, is to become completely passive and to relinquish all responsibility for movement to your helper. This collaborative activity will allow you to release tension patterns that can inhibit movement. The *head lift* with a partner (see text box 7.2) can release tension in the muscles of the neck and shoulders, and the *hip lift* releases tension in the muscles of the hip, particularly the hip flexors. The *scapula lift* releases tension in the shoulders and rib cage. The lifts are described in chapter 19 of Sally Fitt's *Dance Kinesiology*.

Head Lift with Partner

Adapted from Fitt (1996, 433); lifts for other parts of the body are described on pages 430–34.

To reduce neck tension, the recipient lies supine on the floor, and the helper sits on the floor above the recipient's head in a straddle position. The helper's fingers spread wide to provide secure support under the recipient's head. The head is moved slowly and gently to flex the neck (like nodding yes) and rotate it (like gesturing no). When the head feels very heavy, the helper gently places it on the floor. The helper's hands should remain in contact with the recipient's head for several seconds to support it as it rests on the floor.

Somatic (body) training methods such as Alexander, Ideokinesis, Body-Mind Centering, Skinner Release, and Klein techniques take eliminating excess tension and promoting efficient movement as a central purpose. For an overview of somatic training techniques, see chapter 17 in *Dance Kinesiology* or check the Resources section in part 3 of this text.

More Relaxation Tools

Other tension releasing techniques that are popular with dancers include massage, patterned breathing, imagery, and listening to music. Some professional dancers include massage as part of their weekly training programs to keep their bodies in balance. Therapeutic or sport massage offers a variety of benefits with releasing tension at the top of the list (Leivadi et al., 1999). A brief massage for the feet is described by Franklin (2006, 20–21).

Focusing on *breathing* can release tension. Special attention to breathing is fundamental to many yoga and yoga-based training methods (Isaacs and Kobler 1978, 21–24, 46–49). A common instruction in yoga class is to extend the exhale because that is the relaxing phase of breathing. Other specialized training approaches like Pilates and Gyrotonic work include deep and patterned breathing as a central feature of the training method (Isacowitz 2006, 7–9). Using breathing to release unnecessary tension can make muscular effort more efficient. For example, breathing can be combined with eye exercises (see text box on page 109) to focus the effort around the eyes.

Eye Exercises

To release tension in eyes, face, and forehead; goes well with any of the other relaxation exercises, including breathing and constructive rest.

Lie supine with eyes closed. Open your eyes and, without moving your head, look up toward your forehead, then down toward your feet, and repeat 10 to 20 times, getting faster with each cycle, but without moving your head and without adding tension in your face, neck, and shoulders (a challenging assignment). Close your eyes and breathe deeply for one to three breath cycles.

Open your eyes again and, without moving your head, look to your right, then to your left, and repeat 10 to 20 times. Close your eyes again and breathe deeply for one to three cycles, extending the exhalation and using the breath out to let go of unnecessary tension.

Repeat the same routine looking up to the right, then down to the left, breathing deeply with eyes closed at the end of the cycle to release tension.

Repeat again, looking up left, down right (opposite diagonal).

Repeat making a large, slow, smooth clockwise circle with your eyes, but leaving your head still.

After breathing and releasing with eyes closed, repeat circling counterclockwise. Make the last session of breathing deeply with the eyes closed last twice as long as the others, remembering to extend the breath out to help you release unneeded tension.

Rub the palms of your hands together and use the friction between them to create heat. When your hands are quite warm, place the heels of your hands in your eye sockets and allow your fingers to drape over the top of your head. Continue to breathe deeply until all the heat is gone from your hands.

When you are ready to move on to your next assignment, open your eyes and give yourself a few moments to adjust to your new level of tension. Then roll onto one side and through a sitting position to bring yourself gradually back to standing. If you are carrying less tension than normal, see how long you can stay that way before returning to your habitual patterns.

Use of *imagery* to facilitate movement is popular among dancers, and one of the benefits is that it allows effort to be focused where it is needed, avoiding effort that is unnecessary or excessive. The types of images dancers use to inform movement can take a variety of forms (visual, kinesthetic, tactile, proprioceptive), so using images is a skill that improves with practice (Franklin 1996a, 49–55). Imagery can be combined with exercises, dance movements, and other relaxation training methods to enhance tension releasing effects. One especially useful feature of imagery is that once a dancer learns an image from a teacher, she or he can use the image even when the teacher is not available to present it. Another useful feature is that imagery can be used without distracting the audience, so dancers can use it to guide their movements while performing. A third benefit is that imagery can integrate and pattern movement in ways that isolated, conscious control cannot. Lulu Sweigard (1974), Mabel Todd (1980), Irene Dowd (1995), and Eric Franklin (1996b, 2002, 2004, 2006) are a few of the teachers who have made important contributions to the use of imagery in dance training. The Constructive Rest Position is often used as a foundation for imagery (see Franklin 2006, 33–41, for an introduction).

Music is such an integral part of dance that it is easy to overlook its influence on how we move. A dancer's response to and delight in music may be another factor that causes dancers to choose dance over other physical or expressive endeavors. Dancers can choose music intentionally to alter tension in their bodies. The next time you are feeling tense, try listening to a musical selection you find soothing and see if it helps you achieve a better balance in your level of tension. Keeping a variety of musical selections that you find soothing on a portable music player will allow you to use them to influence tension. Of course, you can also use music to get yourself energized and ready to dance when you are feeling lethargic. Going to a class that includes a skillful dance musician can be inspiring for the variety of moods, images, and tension levels the music evokes. Good dance musicians sometimes know what dancers need before the dancers know themselves. When the music in technique class affects you in beneficial ways, let the musicians know you appreciate their special contribution.

Section Summary

Some tension is necessary; we could not dance or even stand up without it. Too much tension, however, can reduce movement efficiency and limit movement potential. Learning to release unnecessary tension (learning to relax), generally and at isolated locations in the body, is an important skill for dancers who want to dance well for a long time. Relaxation is a skill that can also bring you benefits that extend beyond your dancing career to make your life more satisfying.

Complementary Training

The training strategies in chapters 6 and 7 were described separately to make them easier to explain and understand. When training to achieve a particular effect, these strategies are often used in combination. For example, if you want to increase the height of your développé to the front, one part of your strategy may be strengthening the muscles that pull the leg up to the front, the hip flexors. Strengthening the hip flexors will allow you to exert more force to lift your leg to the front.

If your hamstrings (which cross the back of the hip joint) are too short or overactive, they can interfere with lifting your leg in front développé. Lengthening and relaxing the hamstrings can allow your leg to go higher with less effort from the hip flexors. If you strengthen the hip flexors AND stretch and relax the hamstrings, the training efforts will work together to allow you to perform a higher, less effortful développé than either training approach could produce alone.

If you also learn to perform an isolated contraction of the specific hip flexors that work most efficiently at the top of the développé range (iliacus and psoas major) and learn to relax the hips flexors that are too shortened to work efficiently at the top of the range of motion (rectus femoris, gluteus minimus, tensor fasciae latae), you will probably be able to increase the height and ease with which you perform développé even more. Making movements look easy, and not calling attention to the effort required to perform them, is part of the aesthetic of many performance-oriented dance forms.

Training complementary capacities (strength, flexibility, and isolated relaxation in the example above) will often produce a combined effect that the individual approaches cannot produce alone. Look for opportunities to use complementary training approaches and consult a technique teacher who has experience in designing supplemental training programs or a fitness trainer who has experience working with dancers to help you choose complementary exercises. Learning more about anatomy and kinesiology can allow you to serve as your own supplemental training consultant.

Many dance training challenges will require you to change more than one capacity. Training complementary capacities, if carried to its logical limit, will ultimately involve your entire body and most of its capacities. See if you can think of other abilities that you might train to improve your développé. Consider the standing leg, stability at the torso and pelvis, and activity at your shoulders and scapula. If you can come up with one or two more abilities that you can train to improve your performance of développé, you are on your way to becoming master of your own dance training.

Training in Cycles

A topic that deserves mention before closing this chapter is training in cycles or periodization. When developing physical capacities to high levels, it is useful to include periods of relative rest in your training (Bompa 1999, 34). In its simplest form, the approach involves pushing your body hard for a while, then allowing it to work less intensively for a while. The period of relative rest allows your body to recover and prepare for the next cycle of hard work. Training in cycles is used to optimize adaptation, to keep bodies healthy, and to avoid staleness or overtraining (Willmore and Costill 2004, 107–8).

In sports, the convention of a competitive season allows coaches to use the principle of periodicity to prepare athletes for the season and for major competitions within the season. Dance companies and dance training programs that have regular seasons also have periodic changes in activity that result from building to and recovering from each performance. The variation in activity creates a natural cycle of training intensity that may be sufficient to allow dancers to continue performing at peak levels. Dance companies and dance training programs with an abundance of performing opportunities over long periods may entice some dancers into trying to get too much of a good thing.

Pushing the human body too hard, too continuously, and for too long can lead to overtraining, the symptoms of which may include persistent fatigue, soreness and slow recovery from effortful training or performing, poor performance, increased susceptibility to upper respiratory infections, amenorrhea, moodiness, apathy and depression, difficulty sleeping, elevated morning pulse rate, and overuse injuries (McArdle et al. 2006, 206, 460). The symptoms of overtraining are unique to each individual. If you are experiencing several of these symptoms, consult with a fitness trainer to determine whether you might be overtraining.

Periodicity and overtraining are topics that deserve more attention from dancers, teachers, and company directors. Researchers are beginning to study these issues with dancers (Koutedakis, Myszkewycz, et al. 1999; Markgraf 1999). Until more is known about how to organizing dance training to promote optimum performance and development over time, dancers, teachers, choreographers, and company directors might do well to ensure that periods of hard work are followed by periods of relative rest. Arranging seasons with breaks between them for all dancers may offer a reasonable approximation.

References

Bompa, Tudor O. 1999. *Periodization training for sports.* Champaign, Ill.: Human Kinetics.

Cohen, J. L., K. R. Segal, I. Witriol, and W. D. McArdle. 1982. Cardiorespiratory response to ballet exercise and the VO$_2$max of elite ballet dancers. *Medicine & Science in Sports & Exercise* 14: 212–17.

Dowd, Irene. 1995. *Taking root to fly: Seven articles on functional anatomy.* 3rd ed. New York: Contact Editions.

Feldenkrais, Moshe. 1977. *Awareness through movement: Health exercises for personal growth.* New York: Harper and Row.

Fitt, Sally. 1996. *Dance Kinesiology.* 2nd ed. New York: Schirmer.

Franklin, Eric N. 1996a. *Dance imagery for technique and performance.* Champaign, Ill.: Human Kinetics.

———. 1996b. *Dynamic alignment through imagery.* Champaign, Ill.: Human Kinetics.

———. 2002. *Relax your neck, liberate your shoulders: The ultimate exercise program for tension relief.* Hightstown, N.J.: Princeton Book Company.

———. 2004. *Conditioning for dance: Training for peak performance in all dance forms.* Champaign, Ill.: Human Kinetics.

———. 2006. *Inner focus, outer strength: Using imagery and exercise for strength, health and beauty.* Hightstown, N.J.: Princeton Book Company.

Isaacs, Benno, and Jay Kobler. 1978. *What it takes to feel good: The Nickolaus technique.* New York: Viking.

Isacowitz, Rael. 2006. *Pilates.* Champaign, Ill.: Human Kinetics

Jacobson, Edmund. 1938. *Progressive relaxation.* Chicago: University of Chicago Press.

Koutedakis, Y., L. Myszkewycz, D. Soulas, V. Papapostolou, I. Sullivan, and N. C. Sharp. 1999. The effects of rest and subsequent training on selected physiological parameters in professional female classical dancers. *International Journal of Sports Medicine* 20: 379–83.

Koutedakis, Y., and N. C. Craig Sharp, eds. 1999. *The fit and healthy dancer.* New York: Wiley.

Leivadi, S., M. Hernandez-Reif, T. Field, M. O'Rourke, S. D'Arienzo, D. Lewis, N. del Pino, S. Schanberg, and C. Kuhn. 1999. Massage therapy and relaxation effects on university dance students. *Journal of Dance Medicine & Science* 3 (3): 108–12.

Markgraf, Amy. 1999. Periodization as a conditioning model for a collegiate modern dance company. Master's thesis, Brigham Young University, Provo, Utah.

McArdle, William D., Frank I. Katch, and Victor L. Katch. 2006. *Essentials of exercise physiology.* 3rd ed. Baltimore: Lippincott Williams and Wilkins.

Pollock, Michael L. 1988. Prescribing exercise for fitness and adherence. In Rod K. Dishman, ed., *Exercise adherence: Its impact on public health,* 259–77. Champaign, Ill.: Human Kinetics.

Sweigard, Lulu. 1974. *Human movement potential: Its ideokinetic facilitation.* New York: University Press of America.

Todd, Mabel E. 1980. *The thinking body.* Pennington, N.J.: Princeton Book Company.

Wilmore, Jack H., and David L. Costill. 2004. *Physiology of sport and exercise.* 3rd ed. Champaign, Ill.: Human Kinetics.

Wyon, Matthew. 2005. Cardio-respiratory training for dancers. *Journal of Dance Medicine & Science* 9 (1): 7–12.

Wyon, Matthew, Emma Redding, Grant Abt, Andrew Head, and N. C. Craig Sharp. 2003. Development, reliability, and validity of a multistage dance specific aerobic fitness test (DAFT). *Journal of Dance Medicine & Science* 7 (3): 80–84.

STUDY GUIDE

1. What is aerobic (cardiorespiratory or cardiovascular) endurance?

2. Are most dancers aerobically fit? Why?

3. What benefits might dancers expect to gain from aerobic training?

4. What is the general recipe for improving aerobic capacity?

5. About how many weeks does it take to see a noticeable improvement in aerobic capacity?

6. Explain two of the several things you can do to make an aerobic training program work.

7. Calculate your estimated maximum heart rate (MHR) and your aerobic training target, using the formula in this chapter. Show the steps in your calculation.

8. What does VO_2max measure?

9. Explain how you can get a close-enough estimate of your heart rate while exercising if you do not have an electronic heart rate monitor.

10. How can you tell if you are working too hard during aerobic exercise?

11. Why might dancers need to learn to relax?

12. Of what use is imagery to dancers, particularly with respect to releasing tension?

13. Try one of the relaxation strategies suggested in this chapter and write a brief report describing your experience and the results of your effort.

14. See if you can reverse the complementary training analysis to explain how to make your arabesque higher and easier to hold. Which muscles would you want to strengthen? Which would you want to stretch? Which would you want to relax?

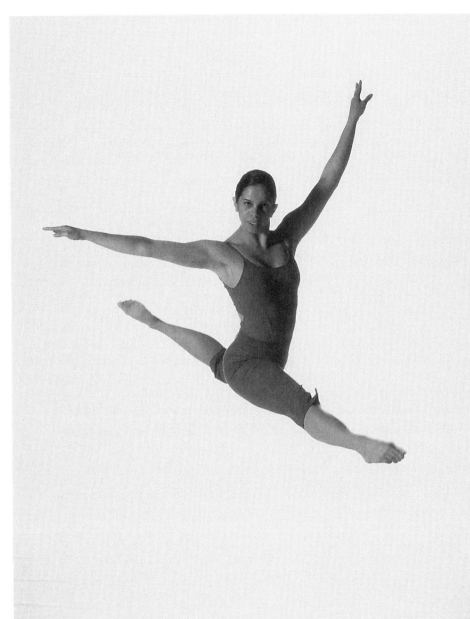

8

Eating to Dance Well

Dancers face the complicated challenge of being healthy enough to train hard and perform well while remaining lean enough to maintain a body image that will get them cast as performers. The emphasis varies by dance form, and the challenge is slightly different for every dancer, but many dancers deal with it on some level. Dancers who are not naturally lean usually struggle with it the most.

Information on eating and weight management can be complicated, and marketing spin and diet fads can confuse the issue. This can make dancers who are serious about balancing health and leanness unsure about what they should be doing in this area of their development as dancers. But many scientists are working to better understand the details of the phenomena involved, and even more clinicians are working to interpret and put to use our evolving understanding in this area.

Purpose and Approach

This chapter presents a foundation for eating to dance well that is based, as much as possible, on established fact. For some dancers, it may be a first step down the path to understanding how the human body nourishes itself. For others, it will be an opportunity to review and clarify what you already know about nutrition and to begin to sort fact from fad.

This basic information will help you make informed choices about adjusting your eating habits and resist being seduced by marketing gimmicks designed to promote the latest fad diet. With a clearer understanding of how the body reacts to food, you can begin to build lifelong eating habits that will allow you to grow progressively healthier and more capable. As healthy eating patterns evolve, and as you experience the beneficial effects that eating well brings you, eating can become just another part of your preparation for dancing and maybe even an enjoyable activity, rather than something that makes you neurotic.

The information in this chapter has been limited to essential details. Dancers interested in learning more about the topic may check part 3 for information on nutrition and eating. If you are primarily interested in building eating patterns that will support your work as a dancer, this chapter will give you a running start.

Consumption

Let's begin with the nutrients you take into your body. To stay healthy and lean, dancers need to consume just enough of a broad variety of nutrients. The goal is to strike a balance that will make all the essential nutrients available to our bodies in approximately the right amounts. Consuming way too much or way too little of any particular nutrient can create problems, but our bodies can tolerate some day-to-day variation. Absolute precision is not essential; achieving a reasonable overall balance is the goal.

Water

Water is not normally considered a nutrient, but anyone who has had to go without it for some period of time knows how important it is. Our bodies are largely made up of water, and they give up water constantly to cool themselves and to eliminate wastes. Going without water, especially when active, can affect many body functions. Even a 2 percent deficit can compromise performance and lead to early exhaustion (Armstrong, Costill, and Fink 1985; Clark 2003, 126). Water is one of the most important substances we consume, and many dancers probably do not replace the water their bodies are using frequently enough. (Note on terms: *water* and *fluid* are used interchangeably in this chapter to refer to all liquids we consume.)

A reasonable target for an average dancer is eight cups of water a day. If you are larger than average, work in a hot, dry climate, exercise especially hard, sweat a lot, or eat mostly foods that contain little water, you may need more than this amount. If you are smaller than average, work in a cool, wet climate, rarely exercise, sweat little, and eat lots of fruits and vegetables, you may be able to drink less. Start with eight cups as your target and adjust from there. You may want to experiment with drinking a little more on some days and a little less on others to fine-tune the amount. Let your energy, performance, and mood be your guide.

Although weighing is not a useful way to monitor body composition, it can be used periodically to estimate how much water your body uses while dancing or exercising (Clark 2003, 116; Koutedakis and Sharp 1999, 42). To determine how much fluid you lose during a class, rehearsal, or exercise session, weigh yourself without clothing before the session, and afterward, before consuming any fluids and again without clothing (clothing absorbs water—and weighs more—when you perspire). Your change in weight is virtually all the result of fluid loss. If you weighed 118 lb. before class and 115 after, this reflects a 2.5 percent fluid deficit following class. A loss of 5 lb. for a 145 lb. dancer would represent a 3.5 percent fluid loss. To rebalance our bodies, we need to replace each pound (2.4 kg) lost with two cups (a half-liter) of fluid. We do not have to make the replacement all at once, but we should understand that our bodies are operating on a deficit until we do. How quickly we need to replace fluid lost during exercise will depend on how important it is for our bodies to be operating at peak levels. The effects of dehydration can include increased heart rate and body temperature, lethargy, fatigue, headache, muscle cramping, and loss of concentration or coordination (Clark 2003, 118–19; Koutedakis and Sharp 1999, 42).

Most fluids (milk, juice, broth in soups, sports drinks, and the liquid you add to smoothies) all count as part of your water intake. Two exceptions are alcohol and caffeine, because they may cause your body to shed water. Beverages with more than 4 percent alcohol (most cocktails and wine) have a diuretic effect; they increase water loss through urination. Drinks with a lower percentage of alcohol, like beer, may have the same effect if you consume several drinks in a short time.

There is some uncertainty about the effects of caffeinated beverages. A mug of coffee or a can of cola, for example, do not appear to increase fluid loss. However, drinking many cups of coffee or taking medications containing caffeine may cause your body to shed water. Products that claim to give you energy, help you lose weight, or help you stay awake usually contain caffeine or a similar substance and may have a diuretic effect.

We suggest counting only your first 12 ounces of caffeinated and alcoholic beverages toward your daily fluid quota. If you drink a lot of either, consider increasing your fluid quota to compensate for possible diuretic effects. A nutritionist will be able help you determine how much to add, or you can do your own experimenting to see whether adding water to your daily quota improves your energy, performance, and mood. Un-caffeinated soft drinks may be counted toward your fluid quota but because many of these drinks contain lots of refined sugar, you may want to limit them. Substituting water, a calorie-free refreshment, and fruit, which contains a variety of useful nutrients, is a good alternative for dancers.

If you currently drink too little water, learning to consume more may require a special effort. One step you can take is to drink two cups of water when you get up in the morning. Our bodies use and lose water continuously through perspiration and urination, so our fluid level is diminished by morning. Drinking two cups of water in the morning will replenish much of the fluid lost overnight.

Another way to increase water consumption is to always have water handy. Carrying a water bottle in your dance bag and keeping it close by during class will make it easier to keep drinking as you go through your day. Having a glass of water on your desk while reading or working at the computer will also make drinking enough water easier. Thirst is not a sensitive indicator of dehydration, so do not wait until you are thirsty to begin replacing lost fluid (Clark 2003, 117; Wilmore and Costill 2004, 431). Since your body will use more water when it is active, drink more water just before, during, and after the most active periods of your day. By replacing water as you lose it, you can minimize the effects of dehydration.

Here are some more ideas for increasing fluid intake:

• Add lemon, lime or other flavored extracts to your water.
• Perk up your glass of milk with vanilla, malt or chocolate flavoring.
• Have a sports drink instead of a soda for one-third fewer calories.
• Add soup to your menu.
• Make instant iced tea* and add raspberry flavoring.
• Use instant* or weakly brewed* coffee to make iced coffee or add vanilla flavoring.
* These contain less caffeine.

Keeping track of how much you drink every day can be tedious and is probably unnecessary, but checking periodically to see how much water you consume in a average day can help you keep your body well hydrated. Pouring all of the water you drink from a pre-measured container (a two-liter soda bottle is close enough to eight cups) is one way to get an estimate. Try to drink about the same amount as you do on other days so your assessment will be a good estimate of what you are drinking normally. Of course, you will need to add an estimate for the other fluids you consume that are not poured from your container.

Filling a bottle in the morning and challenging yourself to finish it by the end of the day is also a good way to drink enough water. If a two-liter bottle is too bulky for your mobile lifestyle, fill a one-liter bottle in the morning and finish it before lunch, then fill it again and finish it by the end of the day. Having a clear and simple goal and an easy-to-read indicator will help you to keep drinking and to feel a sense of accomplishment when you succeed. If your goal is too hard, ask a nutritionist for help. You may be trying to drink too much.

If this approach requires too much planning, you might just sit down at the end of a normal day and estimate how much water and other fluids you consumed. Do your best to recall every sip. If you think your estimate is incomplete, repeat the exercise the next day. Your recall efforts one night will help you notice the fluids you consume the following day. One useful indicator of hydration is urine color and odor. If your urine is dark and has a strong odor, you are probably not drinking enough water. However, some vitamins and other supplements can have a similar effect. So, if in doubt, ask a nutritionist.

Protein

Our bodies need protein to grow and to stay healthy. Protein is used to build and repair body tissues like bone, muscle, and skin, so it is especially important when we are still growing, recovering from an injury, or recovering from a stressful week of training, rehearsals, and performing. Our bodies also need protein to make blood, hormones, and antibodies. Because of its role in building body tissues, protein is often called the building block of life.

Good sources of protein are fish and poultry without the skin, lean red meats, eggs, low-fat milk, yogurt, cheese, nuts, and nut butters. Useful protein can also be formed by eating grains and legumes (rice and beans, for example) together. When eaten during the same day (if not the same meal), they provide the complement of amino acids our bodies need to use the protein. Animal sources of protein already contain all the essential amino acids, those our bodies cannot produce themselves. Check the "Nutrition Facts" table on food packages to find the protein content of the foods you buy. Foods that contain five or more grams of protein per serving are good sources, especially for dancers who are vegetarians.

You can use table 8.1 to estimate the amount of protein you need to make available to your body daily. This table is calibrated to the needs of an average dancer. If you exercise a lot more or less than other dancers or if your metabolism is different from other dancers, ask a nutritionist to help you adapt the recommended amount to your individual circumstances. Remember that your body uses protein for healing, so if you are recovering from an injury or illness, eat a few extra grams of protein each day.

Using your weight to determine which row to use in table 8.1 will get you close to your nutrient targets. For greater precision, use the calorie

Table 8.1. Daily Nutrient Targets for Dancers

Weight pounds	Alt. Weight kilograms	Total calories	Carb[a] grams	Protein[a] gm	Fat[a] gm	Fiber gm	Water cups	Calcium milligrams	Iron[b] mg	Zinc mg
70	32	1588	238	60	44	20	8	1200	15	12
75	34	1627	244	61	45	20	8	1200	15	12
80	36	1665	250	62	46	20	8	1200	15	12
85	38	1704	256	64	47	20	8	1200	15	12
90	41	1743	261	65	48	20	8	1200	15	12
95	43	1782	267	67	49	20	8	1200	15	12
100	45	1821	273	68	51	20	8	1200	15	12
105	47	1860	279	70	52	20	8	1200	15	12
110	50	1898	285	71	53	20	8	1200	15	12
115	52	1937	291	73	54	20	8	1200	15	12
120	54	1976	296	74	55	20	8	1200	15	12
125	56	2015	302	76	56	20	8	1200	15	12
130	59	2054	308	77	57	20	8	1200	15	12
135	61	2092	314	78	58	20	8	1200	15	12
140	63	2131	320	80	59	20	8	1200	15	12
145	65	2170	326	81	60	20	8	1200	15	12
150	68	2209	331	83	61	20	8	1200	15	12
155	70	2248	337	84	62	20	8	1200	15	12
160	72	2287	343	86	64	20	8	1200	15	12
165	74	2325	349	87	65	20	8	1200	15	12
170	77	2364	355	89	66	20	8	1200	15	12
175	79	2403	360	90	67	20	8	1200	15	12
180	81	2442	366	92	68	20	8	1200	15	12

Source: Adapted from *The Dancer's Diet*, a booklet for young dancers written as part of a master's thesis by Andrea Jensen(Matich) (1998), University of Utah; based on 1985 World Health Organization guidelines.
[a] Macro-nutrient proportions (percentage of total kcal.): 60 percent carbohydrate, 15 percent protein, and 25 percent fat.
[b] Male dancers can get by with as little as 10 mg of iron, but 15 mg will not hurt.

calculator in table 8.2 or 8.3 to determine the number of calories you need to maintain your current body weight, and use that number to find a row closest to your daily calorie needs.

While getting enough protein is important, getting more than enough is not better, especially for dancers. If we consume more protein than our bodies need, the excess may get stored as fat. Eating too much protein can also stress your body systems, so aim for the target amount. If you feel you need to eat a lot more protein than the amount recommended in table 8.1, please consult a nutritionist.

Table 8.2 - Daily Kcal Targets for Dancers　　　　　　　　　　　　**Females**

Women's Formula - Benedict-Harris　　　　　　(Follow manual calculation instructions)

Base calories					655	(same for all women)
Weight in Pounds	_____	x	4.3	=	_____	(multiply weight by 4.3)
				+		
Height in Inches	_____	x	4.7	=	_____	(multiply height by 4.7)
			Sum	=	_____	(add results above)
				-		
Age in Years	_____	x	4.7	=	_____	(multiply age by 4.7)
Resting Metabolic Rate (RMR)					_____	(subtract line above from sum)
Extra Kcals for low activity days (add 30% of RMR)					_____	(multiply RMR by .30)
Kcal Target (low activity days)					_____	(add line above to RMR)
Extra Kcals for high activity days (add 40% of RMR)					_____	(multiply RMR by .40)
Kcal Target (high activity days)					_____	(add line above to RMR)

Sample Calculation - Females

Base calories					655	
Weight in Pounds	110	x	4.3	=	482	
Height in Inches	64	x	4.7	=	301	
			Sum	=	1437	
Age in Years	18	x	4.7	=	85	
				-		
Resting Metabolic Rate (RMR)					1353	1353
Extra Kcals for low activity days (add 30% of RMR)					406	
Kcal Target (low activity)					**1759**	
Extra Kcals for high activity days (add 40% of RMR)						541
Kcal Target (high activity)						**1894**

Table 8.3 - Daily Kcal Targets for Dancers

Males

Men's Formula - Benedict-Harris   (Follow manual calculation instructions)

Base calories					66	(same for all men)
Weight in Pounds	_____	x	6.3	=	_____	(multiply weight 6.3)
				+		
Height in Inches	_____	x	12.7	=	_____	(multiply height by 12.7)
			Sum	=	_____	(add results above)
				-		
Age in Years	_____	x	6.8	=	_____	(multiply age by 6.8)
Resting Metabolic Rate (RMR)					_____	(subtract line above from sum)
Extra Kcals for low activity days (add 30% of RMR)					_____	(multiply RMR by .30)
Kcal Target (low activity days)					_____	(add line above to RMR)
Extra Kcals for high activity days (add 40% of RMR)					_____	(multiply RMR by .40)
Kcal Target (high activity days)					_____	(add line above to RMR)

Sample Calculation - Males

Base calories					66	
Weight in Pounds	170	x	6.3	=	1071	
Height in Inches	71	x	12.7	=	902	
			Sum	=	2039	
Age in Years	25	x	6.8	=	170	
				-		
Resting Metabolic Rate (RMR)					1869	1869
Extra Kcals for low activity days (add 30% of RMR)					561	
Kcal Target (low activity)					**2429**	
Extra Kcals for high activity days (add 40% of RMR)						747
Kcal Target (high activity)						**2616**

Fat

Fat has a bad reputation in dance circles, but we need to consume fat for our bodies to stay healthy. Our bodies use fat to insulate and cushion organs and nerves, to make hormones, to carry some vitamins to areas where they are used, and to store energy. Consuming the right amount of fat will not make us fat. But because fat contains more than twice as many calories as other foods, we have to be careful not to eat too much.

While dancers often have to make a special effort to get enough protein, most dancers have to be careful not to get too much fat. One way to reduce your risk of eating too much fat is to choose your sources carefully. Healthy sources of fat are low-fat dairy products like yogurt and cheese and lean red meats and poultry (notice that these foods also provide your body with protein). Foods that are especially high in fat (hamburgers, fried foods, potato chips, ice cream) should be eaten only in limited quantities by dancers who want to maintain lean and healthy bodies.

You will notice in table 8.1 that the target quantities for fat are smaller than for the other food types. Fats should make up about one-sixth of the food on our plates at meals. However, many of the fatty foods we eat are snacks, so they are often overlooked when we think about what we eat. Human bodies appear to have evolved to crave fatty foods at a time when fats were harder to get. Now that fats are used generously, especially in processed foods, we have to moderate our tendency to eat more fat than we actually need.

Carbohydrates

Complex carbohydrates are the foods best designed to provide the sustained energy dancers need to train, rehearse, and perform at peak levels for long periods (Clark 2003, 6; Wilmore and Costill 2004, 407–9). Complex carbohydrates are easily converted into glucose and glycogen, which are used to create the fuel muscles need to function. Because complex carbohydrates are digested and absorbed relatively slowly, they provide a continuous stream of energy that is well suited to dancers' energy needs. Foods that are good sources of complex carbohydrates include bread, pasta, rice, and vegetables. The ideal sources for dancers are those that contain lots of micronutrients (vitamins, minerals, and fiber). By eating nutrient-dense complex carbohydrates, we can get nutrients plus fuel with each bite of food, and that will help us stay healthy and full of energy.

Table sugar, honey, and corn syrup (a sweetener commonly added to processed foods) are simple carbohydrates. Our bodies can use them to create muscle fuel. However, because they require so little digestion, simple carbohydrates tend to create an energy spike that our bodies react to suppress, and this can result in large swings in energy level (Clark 2003, 104). This makes simple carbohydrates less than ideal for supplying the continuous source of energy that dancers need. In addition, foods that contain lots of sugar provide relatively few other nutrients, so they are considered nutrient-poor or even empty calories. Dancers need to be sure the food they eat for energy provides other nutrients that keep bodies healthy.

Whole fruits deserve special consideration. While the calories in whole fruits come mostly in the form of simple carbohydrates, eating a piece of fruit is not the same as eating refined sugar. Fruits are packed with essential vitamins and minerals, which make them nutrient-dense. Fruits are also a good source of fiber, and many are high in water content. Including oranges, melon, apples, berries, and other fruits in your meals and snacks will add nutritional impact to your diet.

More than half of the food on our plates at meals should be complex carbohydrates. Check your recommended amount in table 8.1.

Minerals, Vitamins, and Fiber

Several other nutrients work with those described above to keep our bodies healthy. We need them in much smaller quantities, so they are called micronutrients. Without them, critical body processes would be compromised, making our bodies function less effectively in both the short run and the long run.

Calcium, iron, potassium, and zinc are micronutrients dancers should look for in the foods they consume. Getting an adequate supply of these micronutrients will normally result in a reasonable balance of other vitamins and minerals. Dancers also need to consume enough fibrous foods to keep their digestive systems working properly. Probably the best way to ensure you are getting enough of all the essential micronutrients is to eat a variety of nutrient-dense foods. Some good sources are low-fat dairy products, lean meats, beans, tofu, broccoli, green leafy vegetables, potatoes, tomatoes, oranges, and bananas. In fact, most fresh fruits and vegetables are good sources of minerals, vitamins, and fiber. If you worry that you may have a specific deficiency, ask a nutritionist for help. If you are a college student, your student health center should be able to schedule a consultation with a nutritionist, and the visit may be covered by your student activity fee. Dancers training elsewhere might ask their program directors for a referral to a nutritionist who specializes in working with dancers and athletes. You can also use a food intake analysis program, like the one available online at

<www.mypyramid.gov> to see where your current eating habits might be leaving you short.

There is no scientific evidence to suggest that vitamin and mineral supplements can correct for not eating a variety of healthy foods. However, many dancers take supplements, especially when restricting calories to modify body composition, to ensure they are getting the minimum amounts of key micronutrients their bodies need. If you decide to use supplements, avoid mega-doses of individual vitamins and minerals, which can create a toxic reaction. Instead, choose a multiple vitamin and mineral compound that supplies 100 percent of the recommended dietary allowances (RDA). In any case, do not make the mistake of thinking that eating vitamins will substitute for eating a variety of nutrient-dense foods; it cannot.

Body Composition

The tissues in our bodies that take up the most space are organs, bones, muscles, and fat. We want to give the first three types whatever space they need to function effectively. The body tissue many dancers want to manage is fat. Having the right amount will give our bodies lines that are aesthetically pleasing, although the preferred amount will differ by company and choreographer. Carrying too little or too much fat can also compromise our health and put us at risk for injury. The goal in body composition, then, is to have the right amount of fat for our own body.

Percent body fat (%BF) is a measurement of the proportion of fatty tissue to our whole body mass. The %BF for professional ballet dancers ranges in the mid- to upper teens for females and the upper single digits for males (Chmelar and Fitt 1990, 9; Cohen, Segal, Witriol, and McArdle 1982). This means that, for the ballet dancers measured in these studies, an average of 10–20 percent of their body tissue consists of fat. These ranges are well below the average for the general population and below the averages for many other dancers and athletes. In fact, many dancers would not be able to keep their bodies healthy if their %BF were in this range. In addition, when dancers diet for an extended period to reduce %BF, they risk hormonal and menstrual dysfunction, decreased bone density, injury, and illness (Otis and Goldingay 2000, ix–xii; Wilmore and Costill 2004, 461–64). In women, this combination of conditions is often referred to as the "female athlete triad."

Scale weight is sometimes used as a rough estimate of a dancer's body composition, but it is not very sensitive. Underwater weighing is considered the most accurate way to measure %BF, but it requires expensive equipment, highly trained technicians, and a subject who is able to expel nearly all the air in his or her lungs while submerged in a tank of water for several seconds. An easier way to measure %BF is to use calipers to measure skin thickness in several prespecified locations. The measurements are entered into a formula to estimate the proportion of fat in the whole body. This technique also requires a skilled technician, and it may be less valid with bodies that distribute fat in unusual patterns. Still, researchers recommend this approach for measuring %BF in dancers (Wilmerding, Gibson, Mermier, and Bivins 2003).

Staying Lean

To stay lean, dancers need to burn as many calories as they consume. If dancers consume more calories than their bodies can use, their bodies will store the excess as fat, and each dancer's body will decide where to put the fat based largely on gender and genetics. Spot reducing is generally considered a myth (Chmelar and Fitt 1990, 7; Wilmore and Costill 2004, 686). If dancers consume fewer calories than they burn, their bodies will first slow down to try to perform the essential body functions using fewer calories. If more energy is needed, our bodies will convert other muscle and fat into fuel. Too large a calorie deficit can actually compromise movement and cognitive capabilities. If blood glucose levels fall too low, we experience what marathon runners call "hitting the wall"—our body goes wobbly, and we cannot concentrate (Clark 2003, 150; McArdle et al. 2006, 148). This is what diabetics experience when they get their insulin dosage so high that it clears the blood of its essential glucose. When this happens, they basically cannot function.

Most experts agree that the best way to change body composition is to reduce the number of calories you consume each day by a modest amount and to add a well-tailored exercise program to your weekly regimen (Wilmore and Costill 2004, 466). Reducing consumption by too large an amount can put your body into an energy conservation mode and compromise your training and performing efforts (Chmelar and Fitt 1990, 5). Consuming about 200 fewer calories a day than normal will encourage your body to burn stored energy, but still allow you to maintain muscle activity and mental concentration (Clark 2003, 150–52). Balancing these trade-offs is especially important for active dancers.

Whenever you are working under a calorie deficit, you will want to give special attention to ensuring that the foods you are eating are varied and balanced so your body gets all the nutrients it needs. Based on their experience with dancers, Chmelar and Fitt (1990) recommend a slightly different balance when trying to change body composition. They suggest 60 percent carbohydrates, 20 percent protein, and 20 percent fat. They also suggest distributing your calorie intake as evenly as possible throughout the day to keep your energy level high enough to help you work effectively. A nutritionist can help you develop an eating plan that fits your daily routine and monitor your progress.

A tailored exercise program, including strengthening and aerobic components, is an essential component of most programs designed to change body composition. Strength (or resistance) training signals your body not to make fuel out of the muscle tissue you need to dance. Aerobic exercise can reverse the natural tendency for metabolism to slow down when your body is working on a calorie deficit. Regular aerobic exercise can keep your body's rate of calorie burning elevated throughout the day, even while studying and sleeping (Chmelar and Fitt 1990, 7).

With all the moving dancers do while taking classes and rehearsing, you would think that they would be burning plenty of calories. However, most dance activity burns only about 200 calories per hour (Calabrese and Kirkendall 1983; Chmelar and Fitt 1990, 9). By comparison, jogging at a moderate pace (eight minutes per mile) burns more than 500 calories per hour (Wilmore and Costill 2004, 148). Most dancers need some type of aerobic activity to burn extra calories, and they need some strength training (e.g., Pilates or Gyrotonic work) to be sure that useful muscle does not get converted into fuel on the days when their bodies are burning more calories than they have consumed.

There are some choices to make about the level of aerobic activity when working to become leaner. More vigorous exercise, 80–85 percent of your maximum heart rate, for example, will burn more calories per minute than less intense exercise. If you have only 30 minutes to exercise, working at the higher end of your range will make a greater contribution to staying lean. However, our bodies can convert more body fat into fuel at a heart rate closer to 55–60 percent of maximum (McArdle, Katch, and Katch 2005, 6, 57; Wilmore and Costill 2004, 192). It will take longer to burn the same number of calories when working at a lower rate, so you will have to exercise longer (Pollock 1988, 259–60). As with many aspects of the dancer's training, variety may be the best approach—some days go fast; some days go long.

The information in chapters 6 and 7 and a skilled fitness trainer can help you create a training program to match your goals, schedule, and temperament. With any aerobic training activity, be sure to use good equipment to protect your body from repeated stress, increase overload (duration, speed, frequency) gradually, watch for signs of overuse, and change the way you are working if overuse symptoms begin to appear. You will also want to keep your aerobic training efforts in balance with the rest of your dance training. This may mean mounting any serious efforts to reduce body fat during your off-season.

Transitional Weight Gain

Many dancers say they gain weight when they go away to college. Why is that, and what can dancers do to minimize weight gain during major life transitions? We know of no research that answers the question directly, but there are some possible influences. Anticipating them may help you manage your own transitions.

For some dancers, being away from home and having to make food choices on their own, or maybe even cook for themselves for the first time, can contribute to the tendency to gain weight. Facing the new stresses that being away from home creates, including taking responsibility for selecting and preparing food, probably also contributes. Long hours of studying, a sedentary activity, may even play a role.

The transition from high school to college also often coincides with important developmental changes. From the time we are born and into our adolescent years, our bodies use lots of energy for growth. As teenage bodies become adult bodies, less energy is needed for growth, and if we continue to eat and exercise like we did as teenagers, the calories no longer needed for growth can create a calorie surplus, and our bodies are likely to store those extra calories as fat. To re-create balance, we need to eat fewer calories, increase exercise, or do both in balanced proportions.

Other coincidental factors can also contribute to weight gain: genetic predisposition, changes in training approach, and frequent partying involving drinking and snacking. A nutritionist can help you sort through the possible contributors to identify those that may give you some leverage in managing weight gain.

In sum, transitional weight gain may result from natural processes that have a physiological basis, and anticipating the transition can help you negotiate it. However, it is important to acknowledge that each body is on its own schedule. Bodies make the transition from growing adolescent to maintaining adult at different ages and at different rates of change. You may have already experienced the transition, or you may not experience it until you finish your schooling and start dancing professionally. Your biological clock is just running at its own pace.

Diets

Weight-loss diets are, by definition, temporary. Avoid them, and change your eating habits instead (Clark 2003, 230; Fitt 1996, 447). Temporary leanness is not useful to dancers; dancers need to stay lean, healthy, and fit. Changing your eating habits for the long term will take more persistence, but the results will have a lasting influence on your career and your health. If you are tempted to diet, read one of the nutrition books listed in part 3 to learn more about the consequences of dieting. If you have access to a nutritionist who has no financial interest in promoting a particular diet, ask for help in designing a plan for changing your eating and exercise habits for the long term. The investment will pay returns for years to come.

Disordered Eating

The challenges outlined at the beginning of this chapter can lead some dancers to try eating patterns that are dysfunctional or even dangerous. Some dancers binge on food, then purge by vomiting or by using drugs to cause their bodies to expel the food they have consumed before it can be processed. Others eat so little, or they eat food of such a limited variety, that their bodies do not get the nutrients needed to operate effectively or the energy needed to train and perform at optimum levels.

Disordered eating patterns may start innocently, but can become insidious and destructive. Such patterns among dancers may result from the professional demands for extreme leanness in some wings of the profession. Once dancers learn to prioritize the many competing influences on their lives, and once they decide to take responsibility for the type of dancer they are becoming, they can choose to change the way they eat instead of assuming habits that can threaten their health, their careers, and possibly their lives.

Because habits, once established, can be so difficult to change, it is best to completely avoid dysfunctional patterns of eating. Ask any smoker who has tried to quit, and she will probably tell you that it would have been far easier not to have started smoking in the first place. If you find yourself tempted to engage in destructive eating patterns, make an appointment with a nutritionist who can help you build an approach to eating that will support your efforts to dance well for as long as you want to keep dancing.

Performance Meals

If you are eating well-balanced meals at other times, your performance meals should not be a lot different. You may want to give a little more emphasis to complex carbohydrates to be sure you have a continuous supply of energy while performing, and you may want to eat slightly less than normal to minimize any queasiness you experience when nervous. You will probably also want to avoid foods that have distracting effects, like spicy and greasy foods that may cause gastrointestinal distress and feelings of heaviness. It is probably best to avoid foods that take a long time to digest, such as red meat, since that would divert some of your performance energy to the process of digestion. If possible, choose familiar foods for your performance meals.

Eating sugar just before a performance does not give our bodies extra energy to perform well. When our bodies detect extra sugar eaten as a simple carbohydrate, they compensate by producing more insulin, which can actually reduce the amount of glucose (muscle fuel) circulating in our blood (Costill et al. 1977; Wilmore and Costill 2004, 411). So the effect of eating extra sugar is likely to have an effect opposite the one desired.

Sports nutritionists recommend eating your performance meal two to three hours before you perform (Wilmore and Costill 2004, 435). You may want to experiment to find a lead time that works for you, but realize that if you have not eaten during the four hours before a performance, you will be performing with an energy deficit. Nancy Clark (2003, 149) suggests rehearsing your pre-performance eating plan some time before the big performance arrives, so you will know what works for you before it really counts.

When your performance ends, replenish your fluids and eat the rest of the food you need to meet your nutrient goals for the day. Our bodies restock their fuel supplies more efficiently right after exercise, so do not wait too long to eat. This is particularly important during long concert runs, when performing on consecutive days can make a dancer progressively more tired.

Guidelines

We made a sincere effort to minimize unnecessary detail, but there is still a lot of information in this chapter. Eating to dance well is a complex topic, even when it is simplified. Many of the details, however, do not need to occupy your attention all of the time. The background they provide can help you understand the importance of eating well and motivate you to eat in ways that make you healthier and support your training as a dancer. A limited number of guidelines that can be used as daily reminders may also be helpful.

The original food pyramid posted by the Massachusetts Institute of Technology—<http://web.mit.edu/athletics/sportsmedicine/wcrfoodpyr.html>—and the vegetarian diet pyramid, offered by the American Dietetic Association—<http://www.vrg.org/nutrition/adapyramid.htm>—offer guidance in a graphic format. The bottom two rows of the pyramid, its broad foundation, consist mostly of complex carbohydrates that provide the fuel dancers need to train hard and perform well. The third row includes foods that combine protein and fat, nutrients needed in smaller quantities by active dancers. Vitamins, minerals, and fiber are distributed across the bottom three rows. The top row of the pyramid consists largely of high-calorie, low-nutrient foods that dancers will want to avoid most of the time.

The original food pyramid has been criticized as recommending too many servings for grains, vegetables, and fruits. However, the serving sizes are about half the normal portion size, so the quantities recommended are in line with many current recommendations. A new food pyramid was released in 2005 and is available at <http://www.mypyramid.gov>. The new pyramid does not have the logical clarity of the original, but there are several useful tools on the Web site that go with it, including an online eating and exercise log that will assess your match to current recommendations. Using one of the food pyramids can help you evolve your eating patterns in a productive direction. We offer another set of guidelines below.

Guidelines for Eating to Dance Well (adapted from Jensen 1998 and Fitt 1996)

1. Drink eight cups of water throughout the day.
2. Eat a variety of nutrient-dense foods.
3. Eat at least breakfast and two other meals; go no longer than four hours without eating.
4. Schedule time for meals, and plan ahead to make healthy foods convenient to eat.
5. Carry nutrient-dense snacks in your dance bag.
6. Eat familiar complex carbohydrates two to three hours before a performance.

7. Choose the lowest-fat alternatives at fast-food restaurants.

8. Schedule any body-fat reduction efforts during your off-season.

9. Add aerobic and strength exercise when restricting calories.

10. Don't diet; change your eating habits instead.

Nancy Clark's *Sports Nutrition Guidebook* includes a chapter on healthy snacking (2003, 89–111) and 100 pages of healthy recipes for physically active people. Dancers seeking more guidance for healthy eating might start there.

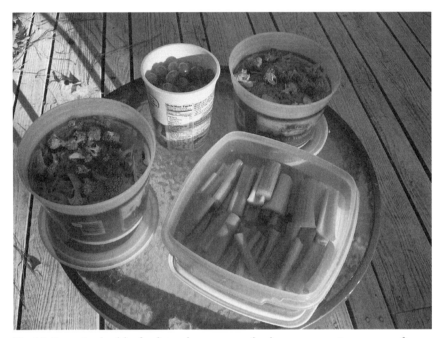

Fig. 8.1. Preparing healthy foods in advance can make them as convenient to eat as fast foods.

Changing Habits

A habit is helpful when it generates beneficial effects. For example, if you learned to drink a lot of water when you were young, that habit is probably serving you well now. You naturally tend to drink plenty of water without thinking about it.

Habits that produce detrimental effects, like eating too many fatty or sugary foods, highlight the disadvantage of habits. This kind of habit will make it feel natural to eat too many calorie-dense, nutrient-poor foods, so we have to constantly resist doing something that produces unhealthy side effects. It has been said that it takes 39 days to change a habit (Collins 1983). While the exact number of days is probably arbitrary, the point is that you cannot give up after a day or two or even a week or two if a new habit does not yet feel as natural as the one you are trying to replace. You may have to persist with some challenging work for a month or more to establish your new habit. Only after an extended, focused effort will your new habit begin to feel as natural as the old one once did.

Caution: Habits can be difficult to change, so use discretion when deciding which habits you allow yourself to develop.

Summary

There are strategies for developing new habits. If you would like help changing your eating habits, consult a nutritionist or a behavior specialist. Many campus health centers can connect you with a counselor who can help you establish new habits. Whether you decide to employ a helper or not, remember that you have had years of practice with your old habits. If it takes awhile to change to a new habit, that is normal. Once established, however, your new habit will begin to feel natural, and it will help you continue doing what is good for your health and your career.

Note

This chapter was written with substantial help from Dr. Mae Cleveland, retired staff nutritionist for the Florida State University student health center. It was inspired by a booklet entitled "The Dancer's Diet," written in 1998 by Andrea Jensen.

References

Armstrong, L. W., D. L. Costill, and W. J. Fink. 1985. Influence of diuretic-induced dehydration on competitive running performance. *Medicine & Science in Sports & Exercise* 17: 456–61.

Calabrese, L. H., and D. T. Kirkendall. 1983. Nutritional and medical considerations in dancers. *Clinics in sports medicine* 2 (3): 539–48.

Chmelar, Robin D., and Sally S. Fitt. 1990. *Diet for dancers*. Pennington, N.J.: Princeton Book Company.

Clark, Nancy. 2003. *Sports nutrition guidebook*. 3rd ed. Champaign, Ill.: Human Kinetics.

Cohen, J. L., K. R. Segal, Ira Witriol, and William D. McArdle. 1982. Cardiorespiratory responses to ballet exercise and the VO_2max of elite ballet dancers. *Medicine & Science in Sports & Exercise* 14 (3): 212–17.

Collins, Phillip. 1983. Water: Do you drink enough? *Mother Earth News,* November/ December, 84–85.

Costill, D. L., E. Coyle, G. Dalsky, W. Evans, W. Fink, and D. Hoopes. 1977. Effects of elevated plasma FFA and insulin on muscle glycogen usage during exercise. *Journal of Applied Physiology* 43: 695–99.

Fitt, Sally. 1996. *Dance kinesiology.* 2nd ed. New York: Schirmer.

Koutedakis, Yiannis, and N. C. Craig Sharp, eds. 1999. *The fit and healthy dancer.* New York: Wiley.

McArdle, William D., Frank I. Katch, and Victor L. Katch. 2006. *Essentials of exercise physiology.* 3rd ed. Baltimore: Lippincott Williams and Wilkins.

Otis, Carol L., and Roger Goldingay. 2000. *The athletic woman's survival guide.* Champaign, Ill.: Human Kinetics.

Pollock, Michael L. 1988. Prescribing exercise for fitness and adherence. In Rod K. Dishman, ed., *Exercise adherence: Its impact on public health,* 259–77. Champaign, Ill.: Human Kinetics.

Shirreffs, S. M., and R. J. Maughan. 1997. Restoration of fluid balance after exercise-induced dehydration: Effects of alcohol consumption. *Journal of Applied Physiology* 83 (4): 1152–58.

Wilmerding, M. Virginia, Ann L. Gibson, Christine M. Mermier, and Kathryn A. Bivins. 2003. Body composition analysis in dancers: Methods and recommendations. *Journal of Dance Medicine & Science* 7 (1): 24–31.

Wilmore, Jack H., and David L. Costill. 2004. *Physiology of sport and exercise.* 3rd ed. Champaign, Ill.: Human Kinetics.

STUDY GUIDE

1. Explain the challenges that dancers face with respect to eating, exercise, and maintaining a body image that helps them get cast to dance.

2. What are the four micronutrients that must be consumed in sizable quantities to remain healthy and ready to train and perform at high levels? (Hint: one is not usually described as a nutrient.) List one of the primary functions of each nutrient.

3. What are the micronutrients dancers are at most risk for missing, and what is the best way to increase your chances of getting them all?

4. What does %BF stand for, and what specifically does it represent?

5. What is the general strategy for staying lean, and what specific things can dancers do to stay lean without compromising their health?

6. What is the major problem with dieting? What should dancers do instead?

7. Without looking back at the chapter, list in abbreviated form as many of the 10 guidelines as you can remember for eating to dance well.

8. Which aspect of your eating and exercising habits probably creates the greatest threat to your career and possibly to your health? Include a brief explanation of why you think it is important. (If you don't want your teacher to read this answer, write, "Please don't read" at the beginning of your answer.)

9. What is one specific step you can take to address this risk this week? Make it something whose completion you can determine with certainty.

PART 2

∞

Dance Conditioning Catalog

Part 1 of *Conditioning for Dancers* described the physical challenges dancers face and ways of addressing them. Part 2 is a catalog of exercises tailored to the needs of dancers. The exercises focus on muscles, alignments, and movement patterns vital to dancing well and staying healthy.

Many of the exercises are informed from the teachings of the pioneers of mindful exercise such as Joseph Pilates, Rudolph Laban, Lulu Sweigard, Mabel Todd, Irmgard Bartenieff, Moshe Feldenkrais, and F. M. Alexander as well as the teachings of contemporary dance training specialists such as Sally Fitt, Irene Dowd, and Zena Rommett. See part 3 for references to some of the work of these movement specialists.

Exercises

Each description begins by explaining the major benefits dancers can expect to receive from doing the exercise. This will let you shop for exercises to match your individual needs. The exercises are described and demonstrated with photographs and followed by explanations of alignment and execution priorities. Challenges and reminders are offered to help you refine your performance, and a list of progressions and variations will help you modify and evolve how you perform the exercises as your abilities grow. References to descriptions by other teachers of similar or related exercises are also included.

Variation

There is more than one useful way to perform many of these exercises, just as there is more than one useful choreography for tendu dégagé. I have described the choreography I use with the dancers I teach, and I have tried to make choices based on functional rather than stylistic considerations, preferring a direct approach to each exercise. Before modifying an exercise to match your individual preferences, try the choreography as it is described to see if it gives you any insights. Once you understand an exercise, you may adapt it. If you are unsure how much modifying you can do without losing the key benefits of an exercise, ask a fitness trainer who works with dancers for help.

Individualizing

It is unlikely that a single set of exercises will be right for every dancer, every day, at every point in their careers. The exercises described here have worked for many dancers, studying various dance forms at several techni-cal levels. While the whole collection constitutes a complete workout for dancers (except for aerobic training), individual exercises may be selected to match your particular needs. I suggest trying them all, keeping the ones you like, and either adapting those that do not fit your needs or substitut-ing alternatives.

Reference Tool

This catalog of exercises is designed as a reference tool. You will probably not read it word-for-word. It is more likely that you will use sections of it to deepen your understanding of how to perform specific exercises. You might read about one or two exercises you find especially challenging and take your new insights with you to your class or workout that day. If you can improve your performance of one exercise each day, your ability as a mover will improve markedly over a month or a season. If an exercise leaves you wanting more information, check the references at the bottom of the description to find another teacher who may be able to help you understand the exercise.

Other Sources

If you find an exercise that feels especially useful, check the "Related Ex-ercises" section for descriptions and demonstrations by other teachers. If you like several exercises from a common source, consult that source to see if it offers exercises that fit your body, temperament, and current needs. You may want to come back to the catalog periodically to search for other exercises that fit you better for a different purpose or fit you better at a dif-ferent point in your career.

Expanding the Catalog

I wrote the 32 exercise descriptions (nos. 5 and 13 each have two parts) in this first edition of *Conditioning for Dancers* to give the "Dance Condition-ing Catalog" a start. If a second edition of the book is justified, I hope to include exercises described by other movement and fitness specialists who work with dancers. Other strategies for producing and disseminating re-sources to help dancers optimize their training are under consideration.

Equipment

To allow you to see the shape of the whole body, we had the dancers perform the exercises on a solid floor. Ideally, most of the exercises should be performed on an exercise mat made of closed cell foam that is as wide and long as your body. A common mat size is 2 feet by 6 feet (.6 × 1.8 meters), but we have used mats as short as 3 feet. A mat ⅜ inches (1 cm) thick is sufficient for most dancers. Thicker mats are more comfortable, but mats more than ¾ inches (2 cm) thick are usually too soft to provide the support needed for these exercises.

There are a number of sources for the elastic bands used in several of the exercises (see Resources). We use Dyna-Bands°, but Thera-Band® is another popular brand. The ideal band size for the exercises in this book is 6 inches by 5 feet (15 cm × 150 cm). If you have a collection of bands (light, medium, and heavy resistances), you will be able to increase the challenge as your capacities grow. If you can have only one band, start with medium resistance if the body part you are training is healthy or with light resistance if the body part you are training is recovering from an injury.

Adding resistance with weighted bars and ankle weights can help your capacities continue to grow once you are strong enough to execute an exercise with precision and clarity. Adding resistance is suggested in the "Progression" section for some of the exercises. Consult a fitness trainer who works with dancers to decide what other exercises might benefit from the addition of auxiliary weight. Be careful not to add resistance so quickly that your body has to compensate by misaligning or by putting excess tension in the wrong parts of your body. Weights, bands, and other resistance devices are calibrated in small increments to allow you to increase resistance gradually, to satisfy the principle of progressive overload (see chapter 2).

Working on Pilates, Gyrotonic°, Cybex°, Nautilus°, and other types of fitness training equipment is often helpful to dancers, both as a way of progressing the exercises and as a way of making an exercise easier to perform correctly when first starting. Dancers in our program have access to a conditioning studio and small group classes on specialized conditioning equipment. If such training is available to you, give it a try to see whether it might help you grow as a dancer. Many dancers become trainers in specialized training methods and use their income as trainers to support their involvement in dance as a performing art. See the Resources section for information about teacher training programs. Sources for mats, bands, weights, and other fitness training equipment are also included. A Web search will reveal others.

Breathing

Different movement forms use different styles of breathing. Moira Merrithew of Stott Pilates teaches that the breath out facilitates flexing the spine and the breath in facilitates extending the spine. Personal fitness trainers recommend breathing out on the most effortful part of the movement. Teachers of relaxation suggest lengthening the breath out to release unnecessary tension. They seem to agree that breathing fully is helpful and that holding your breath is usually counterproductive (power weight lifters excepted, Wilmore and Costill 2004, 260–61).

The breathing patterns described here are designed to facilitate the movement used for each exercise. If you find the pattern distracting, feel free to reverse it, but keep breathing, and breathe fully to provide your muscles with plenty of fresh oxygen to support the work you are asking them to do.

Positions, Terms, and Concepts

Take a few minutes to preview the terms below so you will remember there is an explanation in case you need one later. Reading them in order will make them easier to understand.

Supine: Lying on your back.

Prone: Lying on your belly; may also be done with body supported on feet and hands or elbows (see plank position).

Side lying: Lying on left or right side; may be done with legs and arms in various positions to provide more support (for stability) or less support (to challenge balance and strength).

Constructive rest (neutral): Lying supine with hips flexed to about 45 degrees, knees flexed to 90 degrees, and feet flat on the floor; other versions change alignment at the hips and shoulders to put tight muscles on slack.

Plank: Prone position with weight supported on hands and feet or on elbows and feet (ex. 19).

Figure 4: Prance position with one leg in parallel retiré; done lying on side with leg folded on bottom for stability.

Table top or *90/90*: Supine with hips and knees flexed to 90 degrees.

Planes: The first three planes involve relationships within the dancer's body; the last two involve relationships with the environment. The two naming systems sometimes overlap.

> *Sagittal*: Bending forward and backward as in front and back cambré.

> *Frontal*: Bending directly to one side or the other as in jumping jacks.

> *Transverse*: Twisting around a central axis as in turning the leg in or out.

> Many dance movements happen on more than one plane.

> *Vertical*: Perpendicular to the floor and parallel to a wall.

> *Horizontal*: Parallel to the floor.

Pelvic tilt (see chapter 4).

> *Anterior pelvic tilt*: ASIS anterior to (in front of) pubic symphysis; goes with swayback.

> *Posterior pelvic tilt*: ASIS posterior to (behind) pubic symphysis; tucking.

> *Lateral pelvic tilt*: One ASIS higher than the other; hiking one hip.

Neutral pelvis: ASIS and pubic symphysis on same vertical plane while standing and on the same horizontal plane when lying supine (chapter 4).

Neutral spine: Natural curves of spine at lumbar (hyperextension) and thoracic (flexion) are lengthened but not flattened completely (chapter 4).

Imprinted spine: Engaging the abdominal muscles enough to bring the lumbar spine in contact with the floor. (Learned from Moira Stott Merrithew.)

Dorsiflexion (d-flex): Ankle and foot are *flexed* so toes come closer to the knee.

Plantar flexion (p. flex): Ankle and foot are *pointed* so toes reach away from the knee.

Pronation/eversion: Arches of feet tip toward each other, putting more weight on the inside of the foot, leg, and knee; called *winging* when the foot is gesturing.

Supination/inversion: Arches of feet tip away from each other, putting more weight on the outside of the foot, leg, and knee; also called *sickling*.

Adduction: Bringing legs (or arms) toward center line of body on the frontal plane.

Abduction: Moving legs (or arms) away from center line of body on the frontal plane.

Flexion: Bringing the distal (far) ends of two bones that make up a joint closer together on the joint's sagittal plane.

Extension: Moving the distal ends of two bones that make up a joint away from each other on the sagittal plane.

Rotation: Movement around the long axis of a bone, such as turning the leg out, a transverse plane movement.

Lateral flexion: Side bending; pure lateral flexion is movement only on the frontal plane.

Torso: The part of the body that is above the hips, below the neck, and between the shoulders.

Sit bones: Ischial tuberosities; bony landmarks at the bottom of pelvis that are closest to the floor or chair when sitting.

Lower extremity: From the hips down.

Upper extremity: From the shoulders out, and sometimes including the head and neck.

Scapula/shoulder girdle: Flat bones that connect the arms to the rib cage with the only bony attachment at the point where the clavicle (collar bone) meets the sternum (breast bone). Beginning dancers often lift (elevate) their scapulae, creating unnecessary tension in the neck and shoulders, and even experienced dancers can find it challenging to keep the scapula stable, especially when supporting their body weight on their hands and arms.

Activate: Engaging muscles that were not working previously.

Release: Disengaging muscles that are not needed to perform a particular movement.

Articulation: Ideally, moving one bone at a time in parts of the body where many small bones are stacked end to end, such as the foot and spine.

Bone hugging: Engaging the muscles surrounding a bone just enough to hold it in alignment and to enhance your sensitivity to its movement. The muscles gently hug the bones without gripping. (Learned from Elaine Summers and Jawole Zollar.)

Muscular corset: Deep muscles, designed for stabilization, that surround the pelvis and lower half of the spine, like a weightlifter's belt. Includes the transverse abdominis, lumbar multifidi, and the muscles of the pelvic floor. To activate, imagine all sides of the waist moving toward the spine and the pelvic floor lifting toward the center of the body. (Learned from Suzanne Ambrose, a PT trained in Australia and New Zealand.)

Core control/abdominal bracing: Activating the muscular corset enough to stabilize the torso and pelvis against destabilizing forces, such as a leg circling (rond de jambe).

Stabilize: Using muscular effort to hold one part of a body relatively still while another part is moving.

Mobilize: Increasing freedom of movement at a joint or set of joints.

Disassociation: Stabilizing one part of the body to facilitate mobilization of another; we may use the muscular corset to stabilize the torso and pelvis and allow freedom of movement at an extremity such as a leg (e.g., rond de jambe).

Opposition: Reaching two body parts in opposite directions to create a sensation of length.

Force couple: Two muscle groups work together to create a specific action; for example, activating the hamstring and the abdominal muscles, which are on opposite sides of the body, can pull the pelvis from anterior tilt to neutral alignment.

ROM: Range of motion; degree of movement possible at a joint.

Reps: Repetitions; number of times a movement is repeated. See chapter 6 for guidelines. Sally Fitt (1996, 395) recommends doing five reps after the burn begins.

Retrograde: Performing a movement phrase (1,2,3,4) in reverse order (4,3,2,1).

Conditioning for Dancers: Exercises

1. Constructive rest, neutral
2. Foot circles; articulation
3. Bridging, articulated (pelvic curl)
4. Spine twist, supine
5. Single-leg reach; double-leg reach

6. Hundred (with dancer arms)

7. Roll-up

8. Lower back stretch

9. Upper spine → whole back stretch

10. Neck stretches

11. Ankle strengthening

12. Dancer lift

13. Curl-off: top, bottom

14. Torso/pelvis stabilization

15. Bridging, neutral

16. Tendu arabesque, prone

17. Upper spine extension

18. Kneeling back stretch

19. Plank support

20. Side bend

21. Side legs

22. Hip rotators

23. Hip flexor stretch

24. Pectoral stretches

25. Hip rotator stretches

26. Hamstring stretch

27. Elevé plié

28. Calf stretches

29. Push-up

30. Relaxation

I like to finish with a standing exercise using continuous, articulated movement of the whole spine.

Exercise 1: Constructive Rest, Neutral

Benefits: Focus attention; release tension; find neutral alignment; establish home base.

Starting Position: Supine with spine and pelvis neutral, legs parallel, hips flexed to 45 degrees, knees flexed to 90 degrees, feet flat on floor, arms on floor by sides, palms down.

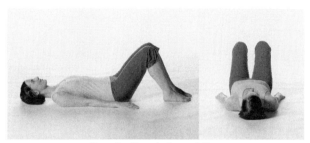

Breathe Deeply In and Out

Movement (30–60 seconds)

Breathe deeply in and out, allowing body to respond.

Release tension in face, neck, shoulders, arms and hands, rib cage, middle back, lower back, hips, legs, and feet.

Engage inner thigh muscles just enough to hold legs parallel (bone hugging). Maintain neutral alignment with minimum muscular effort.

Priorities

Release unnecessary tension with each breath out.

Align knees, ankles, and feet in the same vertical planes as hip joints (perfect parallel).

Align both ASIS and pubic symphysis on same horizontal plane (parallel to floor; chapter 4).

Use just enough muscular effort to maintain neutral alignment.

Challenges and Reminders

Allow all natural curves of the spine to lengthen but not disappear.

Allow shoulder blades and lower ribs to drift toward floor without pushing.

Equalize pressure on the big ball of foot, little ball of foot, and heel.

Progression and Variations

1. Engage the stabilizing muscles (muscular corset) without changing alignment (also called abdominal bracing) and allow rib cage to expand with each breath in.

2. Eye exercises (chapter 7).

Related Exercises

Franklin (1996, 59–61)
Isaacs and Kobler (1978, 47–49, breathing)
Olsen (1991, 13)
Sweigard (1974, 215–21)

Exercise 2: Foot Circles and Articulation

Benefits: Focus attention; mobilize the joints in the ankle and foot; activate the muscles in the lower leg and strengthen those that control the foot and ankle.

Starting Position: From constructive rest, bring right knee to chest and hold shin parallel to floor, with outside hand lower and inside hand higher, ankle dorsiflexed.

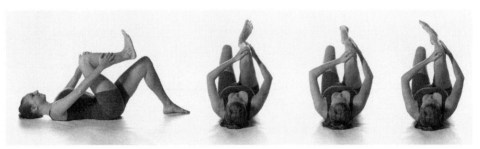

Breathe In   *Breathe Out*

Movement (4–8 repetitions in each direction)

Circle foot to the outside, through pointed, to the inside, and back to the start.
After completing reps in one direction, reverse directions.
Then press through heel, arch, ball of foot, and finally toes; retrograde.

Priorities

Move slowly and continuously through as great a range of motion as possible.
Isolate movement to the ankle and foot.
Use bone hugging to control the movement throughout.

Challenges and Reminders

Imagine stirring molasses or another thick liquid with your foot.
Work through the parts of the circle your foot wants to skip (your weak areas).
Focus enough attention on your standing leg to keep it parallel (bone hugging).
Equalize pressure into mat at big and little balls of foot and heel on standing leg.

Progression and Variations

1. Start with gesture leg in parallel attitude, holding thigh with hands.
2. Start standing with gesture knee folded toward armpit in your 2nd attitude position.
3. "Doming" (Dowd 1995, 44).

Related Exercises

Dowd (1995, 41–44)
Fitt (1996, 408)
Isaacs and Kobler (1978, 50)

Exercise 3: Bridging, Articulated (Pelvic Curl)

Benefits: Mobilize the spine; train hamstring-abdominal force couple to align pelvis with thighs and torso (Clippinger 2007, 56).

Starting Position: Supine, knees flexed slightly more than 90 degrees, heels directly below sit bones, and arms on floor at sides.

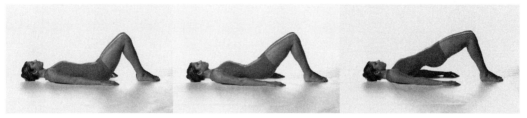

Breathe In   *Breathe Out*

Movement (4–8 repetitions)

Initiate by lengthening the back so much that the lumber spine flattens, then flexes. Reach bottom of pelvis (sit bones) away from center and toward ceiling.

Articulate one vertebra at a time off the floor until your body is in one long line between your knees and shoulders.

Articulate back down one vertebra at a time, upper spine leading, pelvis arriving last.

Continue past flat-back position to neutral spine and pelvis.

Priorities

Lengthen spine, taking the long path to the top of the movement and back down.

Pull with hamstrings to open fronts of hip joints (hip extension).

Activate inner thigh muscles to keep knees between hips and ankles (parallel).

Perform as a smooth, balanced, and fully articulated movement.

Challenges and Reminders

Imagine you have a long tail that someone is pulling between your legs to lift the bottom of your pelvis toward the high diagonal corner of the room

Use tail-pull image to create opposition as you re-place each vertebra on the floor

Imagine a huge rolling pin going from pelvis to top of rib cage on the way up and from top of rib cage to pelvis on the way down

Focus on articulating the spine, releasing unnecessary tension, and inviting efficiency.

Progression and Variations

1. Gently squeeze 7-inch (18-cm) ball between knees to activate inner thigh and pelvic floor muscles.
2. Place feet on a small box, stair, or exercise ball to increase challenge.
3. Add développé or battement from top of movement (see exercise 15).

Related Exercises

Clippinger (2007, 134)
Isaacs and Kobler (1978, 66)
Isacowitz (2006, 45)

Exercise 4: Spine Twist, Supine

Benefits: Activate and strengthen the spine rotators and torso stabilizers, with emphasis on the abdominal obliques.

Starting Position: Supine, pelvis and spine neutral, hips and knees 90/90, arms in T position. To protect the back, stabilize torso while lifting one leg at a time to the starting position.

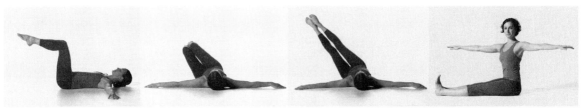

Breathe Out   *Breathe In*   *Variation (2)*   *Variation (3)*

Movement (4–8 repetitions, alternating sides)

With knees and lower legs together, rotate pelvis and lower spine to one side.
Control return through starting position, then repeat to other side.

Priorities

Focus movement on transverse plane (no flexion, extension or side bending).
Insides of knees and ankles stay connected; neither knee slides further from pelvis.
Lengthen axis from sit bones through top of head throughout.

Challenges and Reminders

Release unnecessary tension in chest, shoulders, and neck.
Intensify use of muscular corset to anticipate extension of legs (variation 2).
Renew activation of muscular corset as you return to center.
Do only as many repetitions as you can manage with perfect alignment.

Progression and Variations

1. Start with spine imprinted until strong enough to use neutral spine.
2. Extend knees when rotated to side; fold knees in before rotating to other side.
3. Perform spine twist seated, with no flexion/extension and no lateral flexion.

Related Exercises

Alpers and Segel (2002, 110–11, seated)
Fitt (1996, 401, knee overs)
Franklin (2004, 182, with long D/T-band)
Isacowitz (2006, 47, 72)
Siler (2000, 94–95, seated)

Exercise 5.1: Single Leg Reach

Benefits: Increase blood flow to warm body quickly by using many joints and large muscle groups; activate and strengthen the muscular corset and the torso and hip flexors; prepare to move whole body deliberately.

Starting Position: Supine on floor, neutral constructive rest (ex. 1).

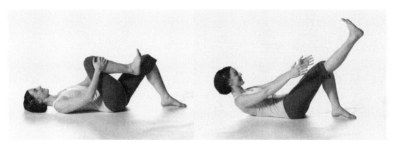

Breathe In   *Breathe Out*

Movement (4–8 repetitions with each leg)

Flex one hip and knee, bringing knee toward chest.
Extend hip and knee to 45 degrees, bringing gesture knee next to standing knee.
Curl top of spine off floor and extend arms in the same direction as your gesture heel.
Dorsiflex your gesture ankle, reaching through the heel.

Priorities

Lower back imprinted throughout: belly button to spine, spine to floor.
Keep knees and feet parallel and in same vertical plane as hip joints.
Equalize standing foot pressure on big ball of foot, little ball of foot, and heel.
Reach through gesture heel to activate shin muscles and to stretch calves.

Challenges and Reminders

Engage muscular corset to hug belly, back, and sides toward your spine.
Move head away from center as head and chest lift in an arc.
Imagine reaching upper back and head into a smooth, curved cookie cutter.
Release unnecessary tension in chest, shoulders, and neck.

Progression and Variations

1. Once strong, perform with neutral pelvis and spine (muscular corset without imprinting).
2. Add hip rotation and hip extension in patterns used in tendu exercises.
3. This version of the one-leg stretch is similar to the Pilates double-leg stretch.

Related Exercises

Alpers and Segel (2002, 181)
Isaacs and Kobler (1978, 54–56)
Siler (2000, 62–63, 44–45)

Exercise 5.2: Double-Leg Reach

Benefits: Use more joints and large muscles simultaneously to intensify the challenge for the torso stabilizers and to intensify the warm-up.
Starting Position: Supine on floor, neutral constructive rest (ex. 1)

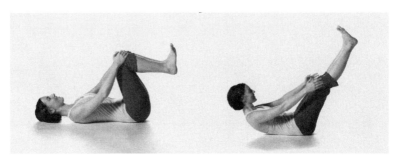

Breathe In   *Breathe Out*

Movement (4–8 repetitions)

Flex hips and knees to bring both knees toward chest.
Imprint lower back on floor and keep it imprinted throughout.
Curl top of spine off floor, extending legs and arms to 45 degrees or higher.
Keep both ankles dorsiflexed throughout.

Priorities

Imprint lower back throughout.
If belly rises, or lower back lifts off floor, flex knee and restart.
Aim legs and arms more toward ceiling on next repetition.
Use moderation. Reaching too low before you are strong enough can strain your lower back.
Doing too many repetitions can irritate your hip flexors.

Challenges and Reminders

Limit work to a level where you can keep lower back imprinted on mat.
Move top of head away from center and toward ceiling in an arc.
Reach through heels and backs of legs to work shin muscles and stretch calves.
Lengthen spine more as you fold knees to chest and return rib cage and then your head to floor.

Progression and Variations

1. Move from single-leg reach to double-leg reach without stopping.
2. As muscular corset gets stronger (over several weeks), reach progressively lower with legs.
   (Use ability to keep your lower back imprinted as your guide).
3. Extend arms overhead as legs extend (Pilates double-leg stretch).

Related Exercises

Alpers and Segel (2002, 181)
Isaacs and Kobler (1978, 54–56)
Siler (2000, 64–65, 46–47)

Exercise 6: Hundred (with Dancer Arms)

Benefits: Activate, strengthen, and increase endurance of torso stabilizers.
Starting Position: From supine with knees to chest, curl head, neck, shoulders, and
upper ribs off floor in a long arc as you extend legs to your working level.

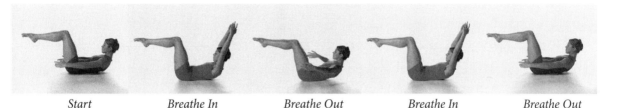

Start   *Breathe In*   *Breathe Out*   *Breathe In*   *Breathe Out*

Movement (5 to 10 cycles, 10 counts for each cycle = 100)

Imprint spine.
Reach top of head away from center, then toward ceiling in a long arc.
Raise arms to 5th over head, then to 2nd at sides, back to 5th, and finally to low 1st.
Refresh spine imprint, deepening long spine curve, as you complete each cycle.

Priorities

Activate muscular corset and renew its engagement with each cycle.
Work at the level your body can just manage with control.
If you lose control or are straining, flex knees or raise legs to reduce the effort.
Move arms deliberately and with control, but with no excess tension.

Challenges and Reminders

Focus most of your effort on your muscular corset.
Soften your sternum toward spine to allow whole spine to make a long curve.
Imagine floating your head on the top of a long, curved spine.

Progression and Variations

1. Pump arms up and down about 12 inches (30 cm), twice per second, breathing
   in for five movements and out for five movements; build gradually to 100.
2. To reduce effort, flex hips and knees more or raise legs toward ceiling; do fewer
   cycles.
3. To increase effort, take feet further away from nose; do more cycles.
4. Add this to end of prior abdominal exercise (to build muscular endurance).

Related Exercises

Alpers and Segel (2002, 123–33)
Isacowitz (2006, 50)
Pilates (2003, 1945, 40–41)
Siler (2000, 52–53)

Exercise 7: Roll-up

Benefits: Strengthen torso and hip flexors; develop coordination to balance body
   weights, especially balancing the head on the top of the spine as you roll up.
Starting Position: Supine with extended legs, arms by sides, ankles dorsiflexed.

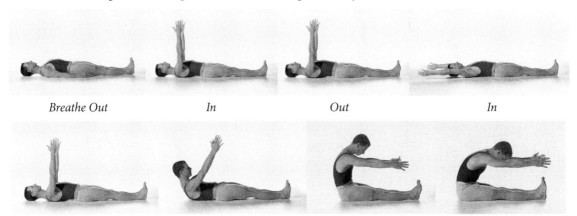

Breathe Out   *In*   *Out*   *In*

Movement (4–8 repetitions; based on Elizabeth Larkam's choreography)

Reach fingers to ceiling, then shoulders to floor (opposition).
Reach arms over head and bottom of rib cage toward pelvis (opposition).
Curl head and chest off floor in a long arc.
Deepen engagement of the abdominal muscles to bring rib cage under head.
Engage lowest abdominal muscles to bring lower back under ribs.
Continue long curl of spine as you reach toward or past your feet.
Roll down one vertebra at a time.

Priorities

Imprint spine rolling up and rolling down.
Work smoothly through the entire ROM without skipping challenging spots.
Lengthen back of spine and deepen its curve as hands reach to front wall.

Challenges and Reminders

Keep head balancing on spine, and lift back of head toward ceiling (rather than
   bringing chin to chest).
Move successive vertebrae under those already off the floor.
Head and neck should reflect the curve in the rest of spine.
Scapulae stay neutral after the first reach to ceiling.

Progression and Variations

1. Assist by flexing knees and pulling with hands behind thighs.
2. Start with arms reaching over head, and shorten to two breath cycles.
3. Hold weighted bar as you roll up, reaching toward ceiling to increase challenge.
4. Extend to forward-pitched flat back at end of up phase.

Related Exercises

Alpers and Segel (2002, 131–40)   Larkham (1996)
Fitt (1996, 401, abdominal curl)   Siler (2000, 54–55, 38–39)
Isacowitz (2006, 52–53)

Exercise 8: Lower Back Stretch

Benefits: Lengthen lower back muscles; lengthen the hamstrings; learn the difference in the sensations.

Starting Position: Long sit with legs parallel and arms reaching toward ceiling; dorsi-flex ankles to strengthen muscles on front of lower legs; heels may stay on floor.

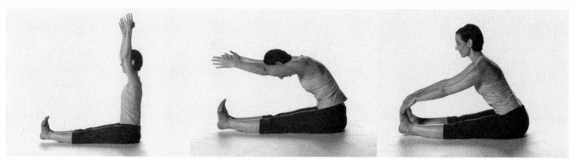

| *Breathe In* | *Breathe Out* | *Var/Add—Hamstring Stretch* |

Movement (4–8 repetitions; then spend 30 seconds in lower back curve)

Lengthen from sit bones through top of head and arms to ceiling.
Curve spine to reach past (or toward) feet (4–8 times).
Lower hands to floor and curve lower back more on each breath out (not shown).

Priorities

Use neutral spine when sitting up; avoid arching.
Focus on making a long curve at lumbar spine when reaching forward.
Keep pelvis vertical to focus stretch in lower back rather than in hip joints.

Challenges and Reminders

Use breath to inform the movement and to release into the stretch.
Scapulae stay neutral; leave room for long, hanging earrings.
Fingers reach in one direction, scapulae reach in opposition.
Head and neck should reflect curve of rest of spine.

Progression and Variations

1. Increase range of motion progressively (ease into deeper curve without forcing it).
2. Add hamstring stretch: lengthen spine, so that belly button reaches toward thighs and sit bones reach away from heels.

Related Exercises

Alpers and Segel (2002, 191–99)
Calais-Germain and Lamotte (1996, 164)
Fitt (1996, 413)
Isaacs and Kobler (1978, 60)
Isacowitz (2006, 63)
Siler (2000, 48–49)

Exercise 9: Upper Spine → Whole Back Stretch

Benefits: Lengthen and activate the muscles in the neck, upper back, middle back, and finally the entire back.

Starting Position: Long sitting position with legs parallel, fingers interlaced with hands on top of head and elbows to sides.

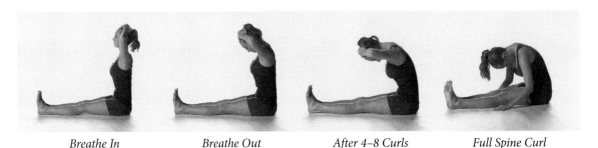

Breathe In   *Breathe Out*   *After 4–8 Curls*   *Full Spine Curl*

Movement (4–8 repetitions; then spend 30 seconds in full spine curve)

Lengthen from sit bones through top of head toward ceiling.
Curl upper spine (neck) forward in a long arc.
Return to sitting with neutral spine on each breath in.
Repeat, involving a little more of the spine on each repetition.
Finish with a long, full spine curl, head to tail.
Relax arms to floor and deepen into the curve for 30 seconds.

Priorities

Involve more of spine, little by little from top to bottom, on each curl forward.
Relax shoulders (scapulae) down, leaving room for long earrings.

Challenges and Reminders

Use breath out to release into each level of the stretch.
Imagine each section of spine rolling up over a pulley before it curves forward.
If middle of back pinches, pause and use breath out to ease stretch into tight spot.

Progression and Variations

1. Longer, deeper curve (range of motion).
2. Pilates spine stretch and variations.

Related Exercises

Alpers and Segel (2002, 191–99)
Clippinger (2007, 144)
Isaacs and Kobler (1978, 60)
Siler (2000, 72–73)

Exercise 10: Neck Stretches

Benefits: Lengthen the neck muscles and release excess tension.
Starting Position: Seated, cross-legged.

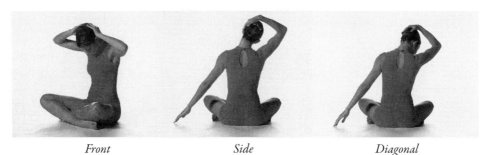

Front   *Side*   *Diagonal*

Movement (30–60 seconds in each direction)

Front: You may skip front if done in previous exercise.
  Place hands on back of head, elbows reaching easily to sides.
  Curl top of spine (neck) forward, leaving space between chin and chest.
  Allow neck to accept weight of arms, but don't pull.
  Increase curl forward on each breath out.
Side: Curl top of spine directly to one side.
  Place hand from same side over top of head and ear.
  Reach with other arm/fingers in opposite direction of stretch.
Diagonal: From side stretch, roll chin toward same knee, head reaching on diagonal.
  Place hand over top and back of head.
  Reach other arm in opposition and breathe into the stretch.
Repeat side and diagonal stretches on other side.

Priorities

Isolate stretch at neck; move ear away from shoulder and vice versa.
Use breath out to release into stretch rather than pulling.
Make curves longer as they get deeper.

Challenges and Reminders

Move precisely in each targeted direction (front, directly side, clear diagonal).
Use top arm to add weight to head, and use the other arm to assist with opposition.

Progression and Variations

1. If hand on head creates too much pull, stretch without hand on head.
2. Increase range (gradually by relaxing into the stretch, not by pulling).
3. Increase duration of stretch from 30 to 90 seconds each.

Related Exercises

Fitt (1996, 420)
Isaacs and Kobler (1978, 84–87)
Watkins and Clarkson (1990, 192–95)

Exercise 11: Ankle Strengthening

Benefits: Strengthen muscles that control movement at the ankle and foot, many of which are in the lower leg.

Starting Position: Sitting with elastic band over one foot; after first direction, both ends of band held together in opposite hand. (Each column shows one exercise.)

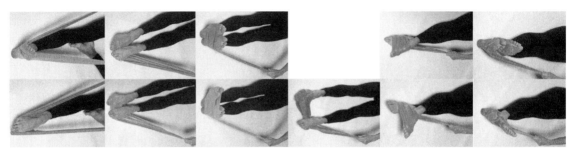

Direction 1   Direction 2   Direction 3   Transition   Direction 4   Direction 5

Movement (4–12 repetitions; five directions; each foot)

1. Articulated plantar flexion (point) and controlled return (dorsiflexion).
   Transition: Step on both parts of band, with stable foot next to gesture foot.
2. Staying plantar flexed, evert (pronate) foot (little toe reaches out and downward).
   Transition: Dorsiflex both ankles (toes to nose).
3. Staying dorsiflexed, evert (pronate) foot (little toe sweeps out and upward).
   Transition: Slacken band to allow imaginary 3rd foot between other two.
   Cross working heel over instep of standing foot, plantar flex both feet.
4. Staying plantar flexed, invert (supinate) foot (big toe reaches in and downward).
   Transition: Dorsiflex both ankles.
5. Staying dorsiflexed, invert (supinate) foot (big toe sweeps in and upward).

Repeat five directions with the other foot gesturing.

Priorities

Work through full range of motion (ROM).
Use a smooth, controlled press into band and a smooth, controlled return to start.

Challenges and Reminders

Spread out band on foot; allow band to extend past toes about an inch.
Resist dropping back to start after pressing into band; return with control.
Make movement smooth and continuous, going both directions.

Progression and Variations

1. Increase repetitions gradually until 12 reps are easy.
2. Increase resistance (stronger band) and restart with 4 reps in each direction.
Progress from light to medium to heavy (pink→green→purple or red→blue→black).

Related Exercises

Clippinger (2007, 344–48)
Fitt (1996, 408–9)
Franklin (2004, 156–59)

Exercise 12: Dancer Lift

Benefits: Strengthen and coordinate use of muscles in the upper extremity (arms, shoulders, scapulae) and torso to facilitate lifting.

Starting Position: Seated with legs extended parallel to front; middle of band under top of thighs, end of bands in hands near chest or waist.

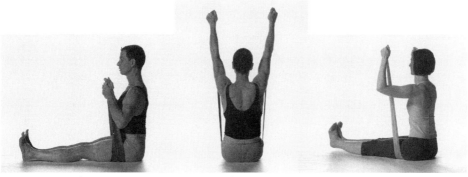

Breathe In   *Breathe Out*   *Variation—Halfway Down*

Movement (4–8 repetitions)

Imagine holding a dancer between your hands.

Lift imaginary dancer directly in front of your face until arms are fully extended over head.

Lower with control following the same path.

Priorities

Maintain neutral alignment in torso, especially at rib cage.

Follow path directly in front of body.

Control movement throughout.

Resist unnecessary elevation of scapulae at top (lifting shoulders).

Challenges and Reminders

Rib cage stays directly above pelvis, without tipping, as arms reach over head.

As hands reach up, imagine scapulae sliding down the back of your rib cage.

Progression and Variations

1. If hamstrings are short (tight), start sitting with crossed legs.
2. Lower hands only to eye level for second half of reps.

Related Exercises

Andes (1995, 166–67)

Clippinger (2007, 438)

Watkins and Clarkson (1990, 24–25)

Exercise 13.1: Curl-off: Top

Benefits: Strengthen upper torso and neck flexors; build endurance in muscular corset.

Starting Position: Neutral constructive rest, fingers laced behind head with elbows wide.

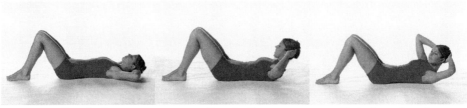

Breathe In   *Breathe Out*   *Variation—Rotation*

Movement (4–8 repetitions)

Lengthen spine from tail through head and engage muscular corset.
Curl upper spine (head, shoulders, upper ribs) off floor in a long arc.
Allow front body to soften into a long, curved spine.
Return to floor one vertebra at a time, bottom to top.

Priorities

Lead upward movement with top and back of head.
Isolate movement to sagittal (and transverse on variation) plane; avoid side bending.
Elbows reach wide and arms follow the movement of the torso, rather than pulling on head.

Challenges and Reminders

Balance head on top of spine; lift head back and up into hands and toward the ceiling.
Bottom of ribs slide together and down to carve out abdomen.
Imagine spine being pressed onto floor with a rolling pin as you roll down.

Progression and Variations

1. To reduce effort, place arms at sides and reach toward or past your feet.
2. Start with legs in 90/90 position to increase stabilization challenge.
3. Add upper torso rotation without side bending.
4. To build endurance, proceed directly to 13.2: Curl-off: Bottom

Related Exercises

Alpers and Segel (2002, 114–16)
Andes (1995, 196)
Fitt (1996, 401)
Isacowitz (2006, 48)

Exercise 13.2: Curl-off: Bottom

Benefits: Strengthen lower abdominal muscles that lift and stabilize front of pelvis.
Starting Position: Supine, fingers laced behind head with elbows wide, legs extended
   toward the ceiling with knees flexed and ankles crossed.

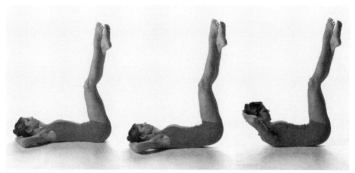

Breathe In   *Breathe Out*   *Var/Add—Both*

Movement (4–8 repetitions)

Pull belly down to reach bottom of pelvis away from center and toward ceiling.
Legs balance above pelvis as movement of pelvis lifts legs toward ceiling.
Return to start with control, keeping lower abdominal muscles scooped out.

Priorities

Focus effort on lowest part of abdominal wall.
Use muscles, not momentum, to apply the pelvis-lifting force.
Pelvis does not have to lift off floor. Applying correct effort will make you stronger.
Lift legs directly toward ceiling, rather than swinging them toward your head.

Challenges and Reminders

Lengthen whole spine as you lift and lengthen more as you return to the starting
   position.
Imagine someone pulling your tail to help you lift and lower your pelvis.
Release tension in upper torso, neck, shoulders, and arms.

Progression and Variations

1. Head and tail reach away from center to create a long curve as both ends of spine
   come off floor.
2. Pilates roll over.

Related Exercises

Andes (1995, 192–93)
Isacowitz (2006, 64–65, roll over)
Siler (2000, 56–57, roll over)

Exercise 14: Torso/Pelvis Stabilization

Benefits: Improve ability to stabilize torso and pelvis against destabilizing forces, particularly when gesturing with the legs.

Starting Position: Supine with hips and knees flexed to 90/90; pelvis and lower back neutral.

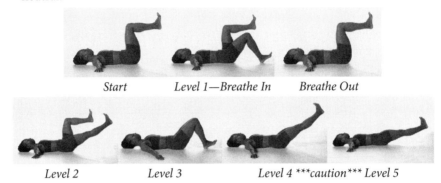

Start   Level 1—Breathe In   Breathe Out

Level 2   Level 3   Level 4 ***caution*** Level 5

Movement (4 reps at lower levels; 4–12 reps at your own highest level)

Maintain neutral alignment at torso and pelvis as legs move.

Level 1: One heel touches floor about 12 inches (30 cm) from sit bones; alternate legs.

Level 2: One leg extends on diagonal 24 inches (60 cm) above floor; alternate legs.

Level 3: Both heels touch floor about 12 inches from sit bones.

Priorities

Activate muscular corset before moving.

Build from lowest to the highest level you can manage with neutral pelvis and spine.

Return to less effortful level when you can no longer maintain neutral alignment.

Challenges and Reminders

Give special attention to transition points, especially when lifting legs after touching heels to floor.

Anticipate force of the moving limb by stabilizing torso and pelvis before moving legs.

Minimize unnecessary tension in neck, shoulders, and quadriceps.

Progression and Variations

Level 4: Two legs extend 24 inches above floor. (Do not attempt until 12 reps are easy at Level 3.)

Level 5: Two legs extend 12 inches above floor. (Do not attempt until 12 reps are easy at Level 4.)

Level 2.5: From 90/90, one hip rotates to bring knee to side, then returns to center.

Related Exercises

Alpers and Segel (2002, 106–9)

Hagins et al. (1999, 546–55)

Isacowitz (2006, 46)

Note: Shirley Sahrmann designed double-heel touch (Level 3 above) to come before one-leg reach (Level 2 above). Perhaps because dancers do one-leg reaching movements so frequently, our dancers find the order above more progressive. If Ms. Sahrmann's order feels more progressive to you, use it instead.

Exercise 15: Bridging, Neutral

Benefits: Activate and train hamstrings and torso stabilizers (muscular corset); improve ability to move with a stable, neutral spine and pelvis.

Starting Position: Supine, knees flexed slightly more than 90 degrees, heels aligned with sit bones, and arms on floor at sides. (Arms are in T position here to show spine.)

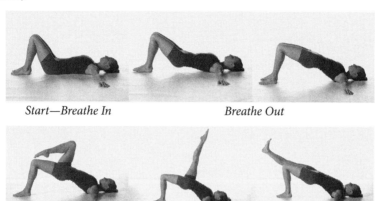

Start—Breathe In   *Breathe Out*

Var. 2 & 3: Retiré   *Développé*   *Battement*

Movement (4–8 repetitions)

Press heels into floor to lift pelvis and torso as one piece toward ceiling until body makes one long line between knees and shoulders.

Return torso and pelvis to floor as one piece.

Priorities

Torso and pelvis remain neutral throughout (no spine articulation).

Movement is focused at hip joints: extension going up, flexion coming down; knees and ankles accommodate movement at hips.

Torso and pelvis move as one piece, like a plank being tipped onto one end.

Knees stay on the same vertical planes as hips and ankles (parallel legs).

Challenges and Reminders

Imagine pressing your heels through the floor while continuing to lie on a moving floor.

Belly button rises toward ceiling with rest of body as one piece.

Back and pelvis should return to floor at the same time, like a helicopter landing.

Progression and Variations

1. Alternate articulated bridge (ex. 3) with neutral bridge (to feel difference).
2. Suspend at top, add coupé without letting torso or pelvis sag toward floor.
3. Add retiré; add développé; add battement.

Related Exercises (All start with articulating, instead of neutral spine)

Clippinger (2007, 215, on ball)

Isacowitz (2006, 62, 84)

Siler (2000, 92–93)

Exercise 16: Tendu Arabesque, prone

Benefits: Strengthen muscular corset and hip extensors.
Starting Position: Prone with fingers stacked under forehead, palms down and elbows wide. Two ASIS and pubic symphysis on floor with both legs extended and turned out.

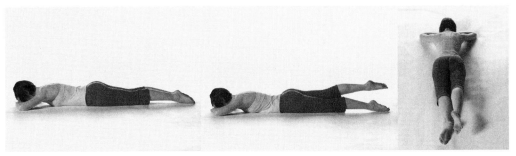

Breathe In   *Breathe Out*   *Stay on Center*

Movement (4–8 repetitions to each side)

Activate muscular corset to resist anterior tilting of pelvis (chapter 4).
Extend both legs, increasing your outward rotation in both hips.
Lift one leg into back tendu (small arabesque) without flexing other hip.
Extend both legs even longer, rotate hips out more, then lower leg to start again.

Priorities

Maintain neutral spine and pelvis as hip extends to arabesque.
Keep both heels on center line so tendu goes straight back (toward ceiling).
Stay open across front of standing hip; whole front of pelvis remains on floor.

Challenges and Reminders

Engage muscular corset to maintain neutral spine and neutral pelvis.
Engage inner thighs (hip adductors) to keep heels on center line.
Lengthen spine and both legs throughout; use repeated reminders.
Release tension in neck and shoulders.

Progression and Variations

1. Add small leg circles in back tendu position, renewing turnout on each circle.
2. Start parallel, parallel back tendu.
3. Raise both legs at same time; Pilates swimming.

Related Exercises

Clippinger (2007, 140, 211)
Cohen (1986, 121)
Fitt (1996, 422)
Isacowitz (2006, 77, swimming)
Siler (2000, 128–29, swimming)

Exercise 17: Upper Spine Extension

Benefits: Strengthen muscular corset and upper spine extensors, develop ability to distribute curve of extension across entire spine to reduce stress to lower back.

Starting Position: Lying prone, legs parallel with tops of feet and forehead on floor, hands under shoulders with elbows at sides of body.

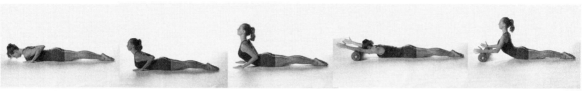

Breathe Out   *Breathe In*   *Progression*   *Roller Variation*

Movement (4–8 repetitions)

Activate muscular corset to resist excessive lumbar hyperextension.
Extend both legs, and press tops of feet into mat.
Lift top of head away from center and upward toward ceiling.
Return to floor articulating from lower belly to chest, chin, nose, and forehead.
Increase curve of spine and height of head a little on each repetition.

Priorities

Focus effort in upper spine, assisting with arms only as much as needed.
Keep muscular corset active throughout to distribute extension across entire spine.
Keep legs together and parallel, with tops of feet pressing into mat throughout. If you have pinching in lower back, turn out and separate legs slightly.

Challenges and Reminders

Imagine a puppet string pulling head in a long arc toward the ceiling.
Imagine reaching head and shoulders under a limbo bar and then to ceiling.
Soften back of body into a well-supported front of body to lengthen spine curve.
Continue pulling belly button to spine to keep muscular corset active.
Reach legs out of hip sockets continuously, and press feet into mat.
Allow space for long earrings, and imagine scapulae sliding down back.

Progression and Variations

1. Arms extended by sides, reach toward feet as spine extends (called "dart" by some teachers).
2. Increase ROM with assistance from arms, emphasizing upper spine extension.
3. Pilates swan dive, breaststroke, and variations.

Related Exercises

Alpers and Segel (2002, 215–28)
Andes (1995, 156)
Cohen (1986, 121)
Isacowitz (2006, 76, 77, 104)
Siler (2000, 80–81, swan dive)
Yoga Journal at <http://www.yogajournal.com/poses/471> (cobra)

Exercise 18: Kneeling Back Stretch

Benefits: Lengthen and relax spine extensors (back muscles).
Starting Position: Kneeling on parallel shins, sit bones reaching toward heels.

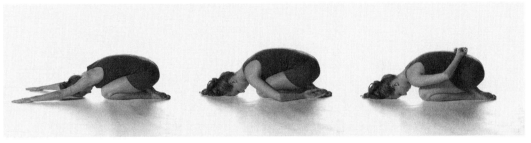

Breathe In and Out.   *Variation 1*

Movement (30–90 seconds)

Curl spine forward without actively folding at hips.
Allow head and tail to reach in opposition to elongate curve of spine.
Intensify oppositional reach a little on each breath out.

Priorities

Distribute flexion across the entire length of spine, not at the hip joints.
Use breath to release into stretch, rather than pushing body into a curve.

Challenges and Reminders

Sit bones reach toward heels as head reaches in an arc toward floor.
Scoop out belly and chest to deepen the curve of flexion across back.
Imagine a heavy head and tail to encourage a relaxed oppositional reach.
Imagine lungs expanding into lower back to amplify stretch.

Progression and Variations

1. Change placement of arms to promote relaxation and stretch.
2. Shift hips to one side and settle into stretch; repeat to other side.
3. Cat stretch and variations.

Related Exercises

Fitt (1996, 402, 416, cat stretch)
Isacowitz (2006, 81)
Olsen (1991, 21)
Yoga Journal at <www.yogajournal.com/poses/475>

Exercise 19: Plank Support

Benefits: Strengthen stabilizer muscles at torso, hip, shoulder, scapula (shoulder girdle), and neck; increase awareness of neutral alignment at and between these joints.

Starting Position: Kneeling with forearms on floor and elbows directly under shoulders.

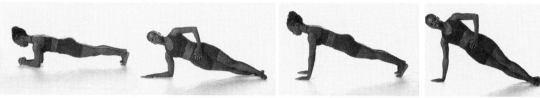

Breathe In and Out   *Progression*

Movement (10–30 seconds, each position)

Front: Extend one leg, then the other, into plank position, with feet 12" (30 cm) apart.

Make one long line, heels to head, with no sagging.

Side: Check to be sure feet are about 12" apart.

Rotate as a plank to face directly side, free hand moves to belly, top foot is forward with weight on sides of feet.

Maintain position with oppositional reach through heels and head; muscular corset active.

Rotate with control through front support to other side.

Return to front, then fold knees one at a time back to starting position.

Priorities

Find and maintain one straight line from top of head through heels.

Clarity of line is priority; stop when you can no longer stay straight.

Rotate whole body as one piece, like a plank.

Keep shoulder directly over supporting elbow or hand.

Challenges and Reminders

Use muscular corset to keep from sagging at torso and pelvis.

Lift head into back space to align head and neck with rest of spine.

Lift rib cage toward ceiling and between shoulders to keep from sagging at scapulae.

Move shoulders away from ears and bottoms of scapulae toward pelvis.

Use oppositional reach from heels to head to simplify the effort.

Progression and Variations

1. Gradually increase duration in each position with perfect plank alignment.
2. Perform with arms extended, hands on floor, directly under shoulders.
3. Lift one leg into small arabesque in front positions (called "leg-pull front" or "leg-pull down").

Related Exercises

Clippinger (2007, 126, 139)

Isacowitz (2006, 83, 85)

Siler (2000, 130–31, leg pull down/front)

Exercise 20: Side Bend

Benefits: Strengthen torso lateral flexors, scapula stabilizers, and hip abductors.
Starting Position: Sitting with knees folded to about 90 degrees and top foot in front,
   supporting hand about 12″ (30 cm) from pelvis.

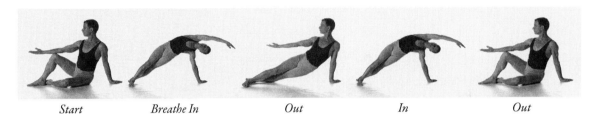

Start   *Breathe In*   *Out*   *In*   *Out*

Movement (2–8 repetitions)

Without bending forward or back and without twisting (pure lateral flexion), lift top
   of pelvis toward ceiling, supporting body on edges of feet and one hand.
Lower other side of pelvis toward floor with control (pure lateral flexion).
Lift and lower twice, then return to starting position.
Repeat whole pattern on other side.

Priorities

Keep entire body in frontal plane, no flexion/extension, no rotation.
Reach scapulae toward pelvis to keep space between shoulders and ears.
Allow gesture arm to follow bending of torso, rather than leading it.
Use range of motion you can manage with control; periodically test your limits.

Challenges and Reminders

Imagine you are moving your body between two vertical window panes.
Activate muscles at back of armpit to stabilize the scapula and shoulder.
Imagine a hook from the ceiling connecting to the top side of your pelvis to help you
   lift and lower with control.

Progression and Variations

1. Increase side plank duration to 20 or 30 seconds supported on hand.
2. Start in side plank and use small range of motion (ROM); gradually increase
   ROM.
3. Change to the other side by going through plank (no rest between sides).

Related Exercises

Fitt (1996, 415, part of "shoulder sequence")
Isacowitz (2006, 96–97)
Siler (2000, 136–37)

Exercise 21: Side Legs

Benefits: Strengthen hip abductors and adductors; develop ability to hold torso and pelvis relatively still while moving freely at hip joint (disassociation).

Starting Position: Side lying with hips flexed to 45 degrees, knees flexed to 90 degrees (Figure 4); head on one arm and other hand on floor in front of chest to help with balance; extend top leg directly down from hip joint (standing position).

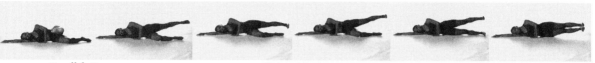

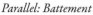

Parallel: Battement   *Dégagé 2nd*   *Beats*

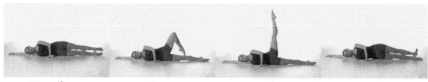

Turned-out: *Retiré*   *Développé*   *Battement*

Movement (4–8 repetitions each phase, each side)

All done with minimum torso/pelvis motion and maximum controllable leg motion.

Battement front/back (parallel): Heel reaches to front (d-flex), toe to back (p. flex).

Dégagé 2nd (parallel): Top leg lifts toward ceiling (pure hip abduction); finish in 2nd.
   Transition: Bottom hip and knee extend.

Beats (parallel, slow): Bottom leg lifts to meet top leg, with control.
   Transition: Both hips turn out.

Retiré, développé 2nd (turned-out): Imitate standing, knee lifts to your 2nd position.

Battement 2nd (turned-out): Imitate standing, leg lifts to your 2nd position.

Priorities

Maintain stable, neutral alignment at torso and pelvis.

Use your own 2nd; unless turnout is 180 degrees, leg will be in front of body, not directly to ceiling.

Use good dancer alignment at pelvis (no hip hiking).

Challenges and Reminders

Reach sit bone on gesture side of pelvis toward your standing foot to avoid hip hiking.

Make gesture leg long, but allow it to move freely at the hip joint.

Progression and Variations

1. Start with both hips flexed about 30 degrees and knees extended (classical Pilates).
2. Start with both hips and knees completely extended (to challenge balance).
3. Side kicks kneeling (Pilates).

Related Exercises

Alpers and Segel (2002, 231–41)
Isacowitz (2006, 74–75)
Siler (2000, 98–113)

Exercise 22: Hip Rotators

Benefits: Activate and strengthen hip outward rotators to improve control of turnout.
Starting Position: Side lying with bottom leg folded into Figure 4 position; top hand on
  floor in front of chest for support.

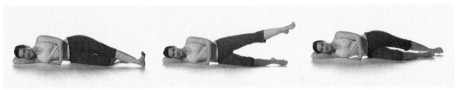

Rainbow—Breathe Out   *In*   *Out*

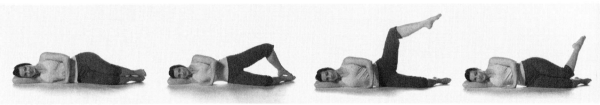

Clam—Breathe In   *Out*   *Knee Vib.—Breathe In*   *Out*

Movement (4–8 repetitions each; repeat series lying on other side)

Rainbow: With top leg extended, outward rotate hip, touch heel in front.
  Trace path of small rainbow rotating hip inward to touch instep in back.
Clam: Top leg mirrors bottom leg; big toes touching.
  Outward rotate top hip, bringing greater trochanter closer to sit bone.
Knee Vibrations: Top leg remains in attitude shape.
  Outward rotate top leg and reach knee to your 2nd attitude position.
  Rotate hip inward and reach knee toward floor, keeping attitude shape.

Priorities

Focus movement at hip joint; hip rotation is the priority.
Maintain neutral alignment in the rest of the body.
Maximize range of motion inward as well as outward.

Challenges and Reminders

Keep rest of body quietly aligned and relatively still.
Leave space under waist so that gesture hip is not hiking.
Mildly wing (pronate) gesture foot on back part of Rainbow; don't sickle (supinate).

Progression and Variations

1. Increase ROM and number of repetitions gradually.

2. Extend bottom hip before starting; knee stays flexed to 90 degrees.

Related Exercises

Alpers and Segel (2002, 236–41)
Franklin (2004, 164–71)
Specter-Flock (2002, 68–72)
Watkins and Clarkson (1990, 138)

Exercise 23: Hip Flexor Stretch

Benefits: Lengthen, relax hip flexors; relieve tension in lower back.
Starting Position: Kneeling on one knee with hip completely extended, and standing on other foot with knee and hip flexed to 90 degrees.

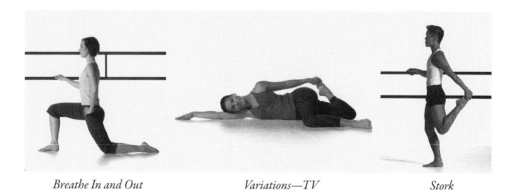

Breathe In and Out   *Variations—TV*   *Stork*

Movement (30–90 seconds each leg)

Activate muscular corset to keep pelvis from tipping forward.
Lunge gently toward front leg to open extended hip a little further.
Activate lower abdominal muscles to limit anterior pelvic tilt.

Priorities

Use breath out to relax hip flexors, without releasing the abdominal muscles.
Keep both sit bones same distance from the floor.

Challenges and Reminders

Open across front of the hip in kneeling leg, without letting pelvis tip forward.
Imagine you are zipping a tight pair of pants to pull belly toward spine.

Progression and Variations

1. Side-lying TV stretch: hold instep of bottom leg and open front of hip.
2. Standing Stork stretch at barre: open front of hip and plié on other leg.

Related Exercises

Alter (2004, 287–88)
Blahnik (2004, 82, 83, 96, 97)
Fitt (1996, 407, 412, stork)
Isacowitz (2006, 151–53)

Exercise 24: Pectoral Stretch

Benefits: Lengthen muscles at front of shoulder and scapula; reduce neck and shoulder tension.

Starting Position: Side lying with top leg in relaxed Figure 4 position.

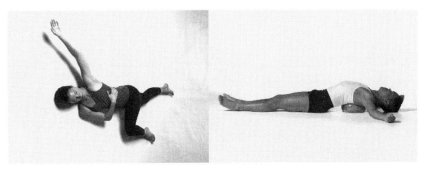

Breathe Out and In   *Variation—Small Ball*

Movement (30–90 seconds on each side)

Reach top arm forward and circle along floor to over head high, back diagonal.

Grasp rib cage with other hand and pull in opposition to reach of first hand enough to lift the first hand off the floor a few inches (or cm).

Reach two hands away from each other to increase stretch.

Priorities

Use oppositional reach and breath to deepen stretch, rather than holding a position.

Keep arm at high diagonal (10:30 or 1:30, depending on facing).

Pull rib cage enough to raise hand above floor so that gravity can create stretch.

Gently rotate the stretching shoulder outward to refine stretch.

Challenges and Reminders

Relax muscles at front of shoulder, and allow gravity to cause stretch.

Use the exhale to encourage body to go with gravity.

If muscles are gripping instead of stretching, leave arm on floor but less weighted.

Progression and Variations

1. Lie supine, with 8-inch, air-filled ball between scapula, arms in high V.
2. Reach back and turn (Blahnik 2004, 49).
3. Deep pressure massage for pectoralis minor (Fitt 1996, 422).
4. Shoulder and scapula lifts (Fitt 1996, 432–33).

Related Exercises

Alter (2004, 292–95)
Anderson (1980, 85–86)
Blahnik (2004, 49)
Clippinger (2007, 449–50)
Fitt (1996, 419, neck pain, 195, 439)

Exercise 25: Hip Rotator Stretches

Benefits: Lengthen muscles on back of pelvis, many of which are used in turnout.
Starting Position: Sitting with legs folded, top ankle crossed just above other knee, top knee to chest with same foot standing on floor outside bottom thigh.

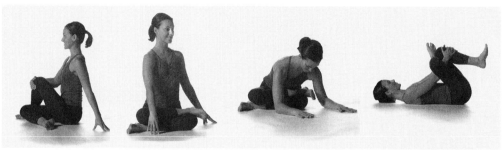

Breathe Out and In   *Start—Stretch 2*   *Breathe Out and In*   *Variation—Stretch 2*

Movement (30–60 seconds, each side)

Stretch 1: Knee to chest, let sit bones sink into floor to fold in the hip joint.
    Continue deepening stretch for three to five breath cycles.
Stretch 2: Release top knee to allow ankle to rest on bottom knee.
    Rotate spine so sternum is directly over bottom knee (and top ankle).
    Lengthen spine to reach up, out and over bottom knee, folding at the hips.
    Reach both sit bones through floor (in opposition to head).
    Continue deepening stretch for three to five breath cycles.
Repeat both stretches with other leg on top.

Priorities

Sit tall and keep your focus on folding deeply at the hip joint.
Release tension and deepen the stretch with each breath out.
Stretch 2: Sternum goes directly over bottom knee.

Challenges and Reminders

Minimize rotation at spine in Stretch 1.
Allow both sit bones to sink toward floor to create opposition for the stretches.

Progression and Variations

Stretch 2 may be done supine if your hip muscles are too tight to allow a relaxed stretch while seated.

Related Exercises

Alter (2004, 289–90)
Blahnik (2004, 70–74)
Clippinger (2007, 227–28)
Fitt (1996, 425)
Watkins and Clarkson (1990, 146–48)

Exercise 26: Hamstring Stretch

Benefits: Lengthen hamstrings; improve front extensions.
Starting Position: Standing parallel, with one foot 12–18" (30–45 cm) ahead of other foot.

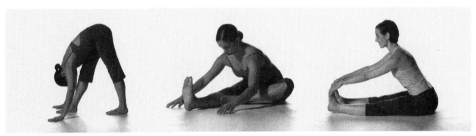

Standing—Triangle   *Variations—One Leg*   *Two Legs*

Movement (30–90 seconds)

Roll forward through the spine until hands reach floor.
Extend spine and reach sit bones toward ceiling to increase fold at front of the hip.

Priorities

Keep legs parallel to stretch hamstrings on inside and outside of thigh.
Lengthen from front heel to sit bone to intensify stretch.
Release tension to let gravity do the stretching.

Challenges and Reminders

Imagine being folded over a clothes hanger.

Progression and Variations

1. Decrease intensity by putting hands on a low box or stair; gradually release.
2. Seated hamstring stretches: one leg, two legs (fits well after ex. 8: Lower back stretch).
3. Ballet stretches at barre (parallel front gives most balanced stretch for hamstrings).

Related Exercises

Alter (2004, 285)
Anderson (1980, 16–17, 36–38, 75)
Calais-Germain and Lamotte (1996, 164)
Fitt (1996, 412–13)
Isacowitz (2006, 151)
Watkins and Clarkson (1990, 140–42)

Exercise 27: Elevé Plié

Benefits: Strengthen muscles that control ankle and foot alignment, especially during elevé.

Starting Position: At barre, parallel, low front attitude.

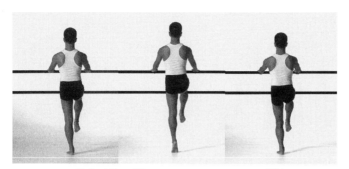

Relevé Four Times   *Plié once*

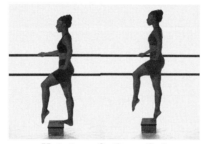

Variation—On Box or Stair

Movement (4 reps, 3 sets, each leg)

Elevé 4 times, emphasizing neutral alignment at the foot.
Plié once, emphasizing neutral alignment at the foot.
Repeat twice more on same leg; repeat entire series on other leg.

Priorities

Maintain neutral alignment, especially at the foot.
Both sit bones should be the same distance from floor.
Keep rib cage directly above pelvis.

Challenges and Reminders

Resist supination (sickling) at the top of the elevé.
Resist pronation (rolling in) at the bottom of the plié.

Progression and Variations

1. Use same pattern on two legs to reduce effort.
2. Use same pattern, turned out on one leg, for variety.
3. Gradually increase elevé from 4 to 8 times, with a plié between sets.

Related Exercises

Andes (1995, 142–47)
Blahnik (2004, 117)
Clippinger (2007, 343)
Isacowitz (2006, 117)

Exercise 28: Calf Stretches

Benefits: Lengthen calf muscles and release excess tension.
Starting Position: Standing lunge, with back knee extended and ankle maximally dorsiflexed; may hold barre or wall for support.

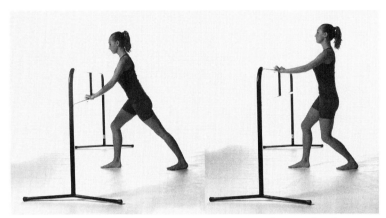

Back Knee Extended   *Back Knee Flexed*

Movement (30–60 seconds, each stretch, each leg)

Stretch 1: Reach back heel downward with knee extended.
Stretch 2: Reach back heel downward with knee flexed.
   Shift pelvis toward back leg to deepen stretch.

Priorities

Keep stretched leg parallel (to stretch all fibers equally).
Stretch 1: Knee extended: targets gastrocnemius (superficial).
Stretch 2: Knee flexed: targets soleus, tibialis posterior, and long toe flexors (deeper).

Challenges and Reminders

Reach through heel and through top of head, instead of holding a position.
Relax muscles at front of ankle to deepen the stretch.

Progression and Variations

1. Stand on stretching wedge or tilt board.
2. Place foot across corner between floor and wall, plié knee toward wall.
3. Seated FHL (flexor hallux longus) stretch (Clippinger 2007, 359).

Related Exercises

Alter (2004, 285)
Anderson (1980, 14–15, 71–72)
Blahnik (2004, 112, 113, 120)
Fitt (1996, 411)

Exercise 29: Push-up

Benefits: Strengthen the muscles that move the arms and shoulders and the muscles that stabilize the scapula, torso, and pelvis; train body to work as an integrated whole.

Starting Position: Neutral standing, parallel.

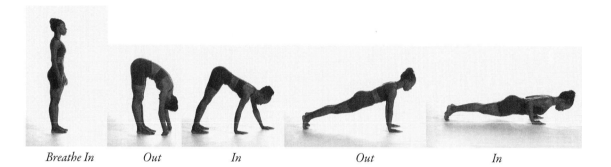

Breathe In   Out   In   Out   In

Movement (3–5 repetitions of arm pliés; 3–5 sets of entire sequence)

Roll down, articulating spine until hands reach floor.

Walk hands out to plank position; refresh engagement of muscular corset without sagging the middle of your body or lifting your bottom.

Plié arms until nose, chest, and pelvis touch the floor simultaneously.

Press hands into floor to return to body, in one piece, to plank support position.

Repeat arm plié twice more.

Retrograde prior movements to return to stand.

Priorities

Maintain integrated plank position during arm plié; move as one piece.

Plié arms as deeply as your current strength will allow; keep expanding range.

Challenges and Reminders

Imagine hollowing out the front of body to resist sagging.

Extend whole body longer by reaching through heels and top of head.

Plié your arms smoothly and with control, as you would if using your legs.

Progression and Variations

1. Start with just the arm pliés (last two frames on right).
2. To reduce effort, start the arm plié from plank on knees instead of on toes.
3. Plié arms with elbows close to sides of torso and finger pointing straight forward.

Related Exercises

Clippinger (2007, 434)

Fitt (1996, 418, scapula isolation)

Isacowitz (2006, 86–87)

Siler (2000, 142–43)

Exercise 30: Relaxation

Benefits: Detect and release unnecessary tension; refresh; restore.

Starting Position: Supine with hips and shoulders extended, abducted, and outward rotated enough to release tension; eyes closed.

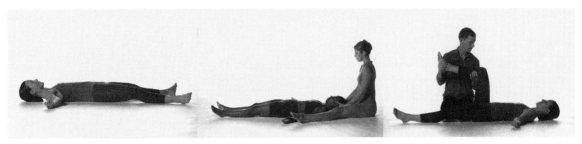

Savasana   *Head Lift*   *Hip Lift*

Movement

Savasana: Let the floor support your entire body; give in to gravity; be passive.

Progressive relaxation: Follow script in table 7.1 (chapter 7).

Head lift: Choose a compatible partner and follow description in figure 7.2.

Priorities

Breathe deeply, extending the breath out to release tension.

Allow floor (and/or partner) to support the full weight of your body; surrender control.

Isolate effort in progressive relaxation to targeted body parts.

Challenges and Reminders

Breathe deeply, emphasizing and extending the breath out.

Observe what happens in your body without trying to control it.

If your lower back pinches, start in constructive rest position.

Progression and Variations

1. As ability to relax improves, seek same depth of release in shorter episodes.
2. Use relaxation tapes when a teacher is not available.
3. Hip lift with partner (Fitt 1996, 430–32).

Related Exercises

Chapter 7, text boxes

Franklin (2002)

Hackney (1998, 61–62, cellular breathing)

Olsen (1991, 21, breathing)

Yoga Journal: <www.yogajournal.com/poses/482>

References

Alpers, Amy, and Rachel Segel. 2002. *The everything Pilates book.* Avon, Mass.: Adams Media.

Alter, Michael J. 2004. *The science of flexibility.* 3rd ed. Champaign, Ill.: Human Kinetics.

Anderson, Bob. 1980. *Stretching.* Bolinas, Calif.: Shelter Publications.

Andes, Karen. 1995. *A woman's book of strength.* New York: Berkley.

Blahnik, Jay. 2004. *Full-body flexibility.* Champaign, Ill.: Human Kinetics.

Calais-Germain, Blandine, and Andree Lamotte. 1996. *Anatomy of movement exercises.* Seattle: Eastland.

Clippinger, Karen. 2007. *Dance anatomy and kinesiology.* Champaign, Ill.: Human Kinetics.

Cohen, Robert. 1986. *The dance workshop.* New York: Simon and Schuster.

Dowd, Irene. 1995. *Taking root to fly: Seven articles on functional anatomy.* 3rd ed. New York: Contact Editions.

Fitt, Sally. 1996. *Dance kinesiology.* 2nd ed. New York: Schirmer.

Franklin, Eric N. 1996. *Dynamic alignment through imagery.* Champaign, Ill.: Human Kinetics.

———. 2002. *Relax your neck, liberate your shoulders.* Hightstown, N.J.: Princeton.

———. 2004. *Conditioning for dance.* Champaign, Ill.: Human Kinetics.

Hackney, Peggy. 1998. *Making connections.* Amsterdam: Gordon and Breach.

Hagins, M., K. Adler, M. Cash, J. Daugherty, and G. Martani. 1999. Effects of practice on the ability to perform lumbar stabilization exercises. *Journal of Orthopaedic & Sports Physical Therapy* 29: 546–55.

Isaacs, Benno, and Jay Kobler. 1978. *What it takes to feel good.* New York: Viking.

Isacowitz, Rael. 2006. *Pilates.* Champaign, Ill.: Human Kinetics.

Jacobson, Edmond. 1938. *Progressive relaxation.* Chicago: University of Chicago Press.

Kendall, Florence P., Elizabeth K. McCreary, and Patricia G. Provance. 1993. *Muscle testing and function.* 4th ed. Baltimore: Williams and Wilkins.

Larkham, Elizabeth. 1996. *Balanced body Pilates mat program.* Video: VHS/DVD, NTSC, Balanced Body. <http://www.pilates.com/BBAPP/V/videos/exercise-video.html>.

Olsen, Andrea. 1991. *Bodystories.* 2nd ed. Barryton, N.Y.: Station Hill.

Pilates, Joseph H., and William J. Miller. 2003, 1945. *Return to life through Contrology.* Miami: Pilates Method Alliance.

Siler, Brooke. 2000. *The Pilates body.* New York: Broadway Books.

Spector-Flock, Noa. 2002. *Get stronger by stretching.* 2nd ed. Hightstown, N.J.: Princeton.

Sweigard, Lulu E. 1974. *Human movement potential: Its ideokinetic facilitation.* New York: University Press of America.

Watkins, Andrea, and Priscilla M. Clarkson. 1990. *Dancing longer, dancing stronger.* Princeton, N.J.: Princeton Book Company.

Wilmore, Jack H., and David L. Costill. 2004. *Physiology of sport and exercise.* 3rd ed. Champaign, Ill.: Human Kinetics.

Yoga Journal. Poses. <http://www.yogajournal.com/poses>.

PART 3

Dance Conditioning Resources

This part of *Conditioning for Dancers* is a catalog of books, articles, videos, and Web sites that can help you optimize your approach to training for a career in dance. Brief descriptions of these resources are offered to help you decide whether you want to track down a specific item.

The items are organized by category. Many items could fit more than one category, and some fit only uncomfortably into any category. If you do not find what you are looking for under the heading where you think it should be, look through the other sections. Perhaps the most comprehensive dance medicine and science reference is:

Solomon, Ruth, and John Solomon, eds. 2005. *Dance medicine and science bibliography.* 3rd ed. Andover, N.J.: J. Michael Ryan. Comprehensive listing of more than 2,000 research articles, chapters, and books published in the English language on topics related to dance medicine and science during the past 40 years.

Because this section is a resource rather than a formal bibliography, I added the authors' first names only if I knew them. Perhaps you will have a chance to meet some of the authors one day.

Anatomy, Biomechanics, Science

Calais-Germain, Blandine. 2007. *Anatomy of movement.* Seattle: Eastland. Early anatomists were concerned primarily with the body's structures and drew them in static positions. This book focuses on the anatomy of movement. The illustrations and narrative comments are clear and instructive, and the topics covered are especially relevant to dancers.

Clarkson, Priscilla M., and Margaret Skrinar. 1988. *Science of dance training.* Champaign, Ill.: Human Kinetics. A collection of chapters by experts who apply science to dance training.

Clippinger, Karen. 2007. *Dance anatomy and kinesiology.* Champaign, Ill.: Human Kinetics. Comprehensive textbook on anatomy and kinesiology as they apply to dance training. Clippinger has served as fitness consultant to the Pacific Northwest Ballet, author and presenter for *Shape* magazine, and coeditor of the *Journal of Dance Medicine & Science.*

Dowd, Irene. 1995. *Taking root to fly: Seven articles on functional anatomy.* New York: Contact Editions. A collection of essays on topics important to dancers including visualization, breathing, and finding center. Author works with two prestigious dance training programs: Julliard in New York City and the School of the National Ballet of Canada in Toronto.

Fitt, Sally S. 1981–82. Conditioning for dancers: Investigating some assumptions. *Dance Research Journal* 14 (1/2): 32–38.

———. 1996. *Dance kinesiology.* 2nd ed. New York: Schirmer. A practical, comprehensive textbook on anatomy, kinesiology, conditioning, and injury avoidance for dancers. Includes exercises and corrective programs to address training challenges commonly faced by dancers.

Fitt, Sally, and Tom Welsh. 2000. *Dance kinesiology demonstrations.* Video recording of 31 movement demonstrations that progress from simple to complex, following the outline of Fitt's *Dance kinesiology.* Available to teachers of dance kinesiology from Dance Kinesiology Demonstrations, Florida State University Dance Department, 202 Montgomery Hall, Tallahassee, 32306–2120.

Franklin, Eric. 1996. *Dynamic alignment through imagery.* Champaign, Ill.: Human Kinetics. Explains and demonstrates myriad ways in which imagery can support and inform dance movement and alignment.

———. 1996. *Dance imagery for technique and performance.* Champaign, Ill.: Human Kinetics. Extension of content in *Dynamic alignment through imagery* with an emphasis on dance technique.

Gilbert, Coryleen B., Michael T. Gross, and Kimberly B. Klug. 1998. Relationship between hip external rotation and turnout angle for the five classical ballet positions. *Journal of Sports Physical Therapy* 27 (5): 339–47. Empirical study of the sources of turnout in young dancers. Recommends using turnout in each dancer's well-aligned 1st position as a guide for turnout in the crossed positions to avoid stress and injuries in the lower extremities.

Grieg, Valerie. 1994. *Inside ballet technique: Separating anatomical fact from fiction in the ballet class.* Pennington, N.J.: Princeton Book Company. Concise description of how to work in a biomechanically sound manner in the physically demanding domain of classical ballet.

Grossman, Gayanne, Donna Krasnow, and Tom Welsh. 2005. Effective use of turnout: Biomechanical, neuromuscular, and behavioral considerations. *Journal of Dance Education* 5: 15–27. Explains where turnout comes from, how to improve it safely, and how to facilitate the use of safe turnout skills while taking technique class.

Hayle, Robert, B., and Terence Coyle. 1979. *Albinus on anatomy.* New York: Dover. A collection of drawings by Bernard Albinus, "the greatest descriptive anatomist of the eighteenth century." Layered drawings are especially revealing as they show relationships, pathways, and patterns among adjacent muscles.

Jenkins, David B. 2002. *Functional anatomy of the limbs and back.* 8th ed. Philadelphia: W. B. Saunders. Well-regarded general anatomy text.

Kapit, Wynn, and Lawrence M. Elson. 1993. *The anatomy coloring book.* New York: Addison Wesley. Out of 161 plates, 31 are especially relevant to dance training. Learn the muscles, attachments, and pathways as you color them.

Kendall, Florence P., Elizabeth K. McCreary, and Patricia G. Provance. 1993. *Muscle testing and function.* 4th ed. Baltimore: Williams and Wilkins. A standard reference manual for physical and physiotherapists.

Kennedy, Pat. 1979. *The moving body.* Reading, UK: Cox and Wyman. A concise text introducing the elements of anatomy, biomechanics, and physiology. Recommended by the Cecchetti Society as background for teacher examinations. Originally published in London by Faber and Faber.

Laws, Kenneth. 2008. *Physics and the art of dance.* Oxford: Oxford University Press. An update and integration of content from two earlier works, *The physics of dance* and *Physics, dance, and the pas de deux,* describing how the principles of physics influence movement in dance. Includes topics such as "balance while rotating," "the grand jeté floating illusion," and "overhead lifts and catches."

Laws, Kenneth, K. Briel, J. Donnalley, K. Platz, and J. Zarriello. 1991. Lifts in partnered dance. *Kinesiology and Medicine for Dance* 13 (2): 10–21.

McArdle, William D., Frank I. Katch, and Victor L. Katch. 2006. *Essentials of exercise physiology*. 3rd ed. Baltimore: Lippincott Williams and Wilkins. A comprehensive reference on exercise physiology. Sections are relatively self-contained, making it possible to look up information on a specific topic without having to read the entire text.

Olsen, Andrea, and Caryn McHose. 2008. *BodyStories: A guide to experiential anatomy*. 2nd ed. Barryton, N.Y.: Station Hill. A 30-day course in the anatomy of the body, taught through movement exploration.

Stone, Robert J., and Judith A. Stone. 1990. *Atlas of skeletal muscles*. Dubuque, Iowa: Wm. C. Brown. Clear drawings, one muscle (group) per page with the origin, insertion, and action described in a table at the bottom of each page.

Thompson, Clem W., and F. T. Floyd. 1998. *Manual of structural kinesiology*. 13th ed. Relatively concise presentation anatomy related to human movement.

Wilmore, Jack H., and David L. Costill. 2004. *Physiology of sport and exercise*. 3rd ed. Champaign, Ill.: Human Kinetics. Comprehensive and easy-to-read reference on the challenging subject of exercise physiology.

Aerobic, Cardiorespiratory Fitness

Cohen, J. L., K. R. Segal, I. Witriol, and W. D. McArdle. 1982. Cardiorespiratory response to ballet exercise and the VO2max of elite ballet dancers. *Medicine & Science in Sports & Exercise* 14: 212–17.

Kirkendall, D., and L. Calabrese. 1983. Physiological aspects of dance. *Clinics in Sports Medicine* 2 (3): 525–37.

Redding, Emma, and Matthew Wyon. 2003. Strengths and weaknesses of current methods for evaluating the aerobic power of dancers. *Journal of Dance Medicine & Science* 7 (1): 10–16. Identifies the unique aspect of cardiorespiratory training for dancers and argues for a dancer-specific approach to measuring this capacity in dancers.

Wyon, Matthew. 2002. The cardiorespiratory response to modern dance classes: Differences between university, graduate, and professional classes. *Journal of Dance Medicine & Science* 6 (2): 41–45. A descriptive study of dancer aerobic capacity.

———. 2005. Cardiorespiratory training for dancers. *Journal of Dance Medicine & Science* 9 (1): 7–12. An overview of aerobic training for dancers.

Wyon, Matthew, Emma Redding, Grant Abt, Andrew Head, and N. C. Craig Sharp. 2003. Development, reliability, and validity of a multistage dance-specific aerobic fitness test (DAFT). *Journal of Dance Medicine & Science* 7 (3): 80–84. Describes an aerobic fitness test for dancers.

Alignment, Technique

Cohan, Robert. 1986. *The dance workshop: A guide to the fundamentals of movement.* New York: Simon and Schuster. Opens with a discussion of the elements of dance (centering, gravity, balance, posture, gesture, rhythm, space, breathing) by the director of the London Contemporary Dance Theatre. Includes basic, development, and jazz workouts.

Hoppenfeld, Stanley, Richard Hutton, and Hugh Thomas. 1976. *Physical examination of the spine and extremities.* Norwalk, Conn.: Appleton and Lange. Reference for medical personnel that dancers might use to understand tests they may undergo.

Krasnow, Donna, R. Monasterio, and Steven Chatfield. 2001. Emerging concepts of posture and alignment. *Medical Problems of Performing Artists* 16 (1): 8–16.

Penrod, James, and Janice G. Plastino. 2004. *The dancer prepares: Modern dance for beginners.* 4th ed. Mountain View, Calif.: Mayfield. An introductory textbook for modern dancers. Includes chapters on technique analysis and anatomy, injuries, and diet.

Phillips, Craig. 2005. Stability in dance training. *Journal of Dance Medicine & Science* 9 (1): 24–28. Explains how torso stability is more about control than strength.

Coordination, Motor Control, Motor Learning

Enghauser, Rebecca. 2003. Motor learning and the dance technique class: Science, tradition, and pedagogy. *Journal of Dance Education* 3 (3): 85–95. A well-referenced overview of motor learning principles with informed guesses about how they might apply to teaching dance.

Hagins, M., K. Adler, M. Cash, J. Daugherty, and G. Martani. 1999. Effects of practice on the ability to perform lumbar stabilization exercises. *Journal of Sports Physical Therapy* 29: 546–55.

Kimmerle, Marliese, and Paulette Côté-Laurence. 2003. *Teaching dance skills: A motor learning and development approach.* Andover, N.J.: J. Michael Ryan. Applies the concepts of motor learning to the learning and teaching of dance skills for children and adults.

Kubistant, Tom. 1986. *Performing your best.* Champaign, Ill.: Life Enhancements. Nontechnical introduction to the concepts of performance psychology.

Magill, Richard A. 2001. *Motor learning: Concepts and applications.* 6th ed. Boston: McGraw-Hill. Recognized classic on how humans learn to move.

Martin, Garry L. 1997. *Sport psychology consulting: Practical guidelines from behavior analysis.* Winnipeg, Manitoba: Sport Science Press. Topics include teaching new skills, decreasing errors, motivating practice, and managing time.

Martin, Garry L., and Joan A. Lumsden. 1987. *Coaching: An effective behavioral approach.* St. Louis: Mosby. Content is similar to the text above but written for those responsible for directing a team or company.

Schmidt, Richard A., and Timothy D. Lee. 2005. *Motor control and learning: A behavioral emphasis.* 4th ed. Champaign, Ill.: Human Kinetics. Describes how coordinated movement is initiated, learned, and controlled. A classic in the field.

Flexibility

Alter, Judy. 1983. *Surviving exercise.* Boston: Houghton Mifflin. Gentle exercises approached with an emphasis on safety.

———. 1986. *Stretch and strengthen.* Boston: Houghton Mifflin. An expansion of the approach used for the text above, with more background information and more detailed explanations.

Alter, Michael J. 2004. *The science of flexibility.* 3rd ed. Champaign, Ill.: Human Kinetics. Thorough resource on flexibility and stretching, including an extensive review of relevant research and 42 pages of references.

Anderson, Bob. 1980. *Stretching.* Bolinas, Calif.: Shelter Publications. Easy-to-read reference book on stretching that includes routines for a variety of physical activities including gymnastics, figure skating, and dance.

Blahnik, Jay. 2004. *Full-body flexibility.* Champaign, Ill.: Human Kinetics. Clear descriptions and photographs of simple stretches. Demonstrators are not dancers, but alignments used are favorable to dance.

Clippinger-Robertson, Karen. 1986. Increasing functional range of motion in dance. *Kinesiology and Medicine for Dance* 8 (3): 8–10.

Deighan, Martine A. 2005. Flexibility in dance. *Journal of Dance Medicine & Science* 9 (1): 13–17. Summary of research relevant to improving flexibility in dancers.

Knott, Margaret, and Dorothy E. Voss. 1968. *Proprioceptive neuromuscular facilitation: Patterns and techniques.* 2nd ed. New York: Harper and Row. Provides background for, and describes the application of, techniques evolved from the work of Herman Kabat, MD, in the mid-twentieth century.

Moore, Marjorie A., and Roger S. Hutton. 1980. Electromyographic investigation of muscle stretching techniques. *Medicine & Science in Sports & Exercise* 12 (5): 322–29. An experimental comparison of three stretching techniques with female gymnasts.

Warton, Jim, and Phil Warton. 1996. *The Wartons' stretch book.* New York: Three Rivers. Describes an active, isolated approach to stretching. Some stretches require a partner.

Nutrition

Armstrong, L. W., D. L. Costill, and W. J. Fink. 1985. Influence of diuretic-induced dehydration on competitive running performance. *Medicine & Science in Sports & Exercise* 17: 456–61. Demonstrates that even minimal dehydration can impair performance.

Chmelar, Robin D., and Sally S. Fitt. 1990. *Diet for dancers.* Pennington, N.J.: Princeton Book Company. A concise, focused discussion of eating and body composition for dancers. Includes a practical and useable overview of general nutrition issues.

Clark, Nancy. 2003. *Sports nutrition guidebook.* 3rd ed. Champaign, Ill.: Human Kinetics. A complete guide for how to eat to optimize performance in physical endeavors. Includes winning recipes.

Collins, Phillip. 1983. Water: Do you drink enough? *Mother Earth News,* November/December, 84–85. Practical summary of human fluid needs and suggestions for how to ensure you are consuming enough.

Fink, Heather H., Lisa A. Burgoon, and Alan E. Mikesky. 2008. *Practical applications in sports nutrition.* Boston: Jones and Bartlett. Recommended by a dancer pursuing graduate studies in nutrition.

Jensen, Andrea. 1998. *The dancer's diet.* Development of a booklet outlining nutritional guidelines for adolescent dancers. Master's thesis, University of Utah, Salt Lake.

Otis, Carol L., and Roger Goldingay. 2000. *The athletic woman's survival guide: How to win the battle against eating disorders, amenorrhea, and osteoporosis.* Champaign, Ill.: Human Kinetics. Explains eating and exercise challenges faced by seriously athletic women, the consequences for allowing disordered eating patterns to develop, and strategies for avoiding them.

Shirreffs, S. M., and R. J. Maughan. 1997. Restoration of fluid balance after exercise-induced dehydration: Effects of alcohol consumption. *Journal of Applied Physiology* 83 (4): 1152–58. Suggests that alcoholic beverages with more than 4 percent alcohol interfere with rehydration after exercise. Caffeine, by contrast, was not found to have a detrimental effect.

Valtin, H. 2002. "Drink at least eight glasses of water a day." Really? Is there scientific evidence for 8×8"? *American Journal of Physiology: Regulatory, Integrative, and Comparative Physiology* 283 (5): 993–1004. Literature review failed to find convincing evidence for the recommendation to drink eight cups of water per day.

Vincent, Lawrence M. 1989. *Competing with the sylph: The quest for the perfect dance body.* 2nd ed. Princeton, N.J.: Princeton Book Company. The subtitle describes the purpose and scope of this text about some dancers' efforts to become excessively thin.

Wilmerding, M. Virginia, Ann L. Gibson, Christine M. Mermier, and Kathryn A. Bivins. 2003. Body composition analysis in dancers: Methods and recommendations. *Journal of Dance Medicine & Science* 7 (1): 24–31. Reviews body composition measurement systems and recommends the skin-fold measurement technique as the most appropriate for use with dancers at this time.

Wilmerding, M. Virginia, Molly M. McKinnon, and Christine Mermier. 2005. Body composition in dance: A review. *Journal of Dance Medicine & Science* 9 (1): 18–23. Reviews research and professional writing relevant to body composition for dancers and offers references for learning more about what researchers have found and what experts believe about the topic.

Strength

Andes, Karen. 1995. *A woman's book of strength.* New York: Berkley. Explains why women need to build strength and not fear it. Describes how to design and manage your own training program, involving machines, free weights, and exercise stands. Most of the text is also relevant to men.

Koutedakis, Y., A. Stavropoulos-Kalinoglou, and G. Metsios. 2005. The significance of muscular strength in dance. *Journal of Dance Medicine & Science* 9 (1): 29–34.

Spector-Flock, Noa. 2002. *Get stronger by stretching.* 2nd ed. Hightstown, N.J.: Princeton Book Company. Describes an inventive exercise program using a 6' (2 m) length of Thera-Band®. Exercises look and feel like dance movements.

Stalder, Margaret, B. Noble, and J. Wilkinson. 1990. The effects of supplemental weight training for ballet dancers. *Journal of Applied Sport Science Research* 4 (3): 95–102. Describes a nine-week study of ballet dancers who gained strength, muscular endurance, and power, without increasing bulk, by engaging in weight training three days per week.

Welsh, Thomas M., G. Pierce Jones, Kim D. Lucker, and Brian C. Weaver. 1998. Back-strengthening for dancers: A within- subject experimental analysis. *Journal of Dance Medicine & Science* 2 (4): 141–48. Ten-week evaluation of a training program that increased back strength and arabesque height and reduced the number of classes and rehearsals missed due to back pain.

Relaxation, Efficiency, Somatics

Cohen, Bonnie Bainbridge. 1993. *Sensing, feeling, and action: The experiential anatomy of body-mind centering.* Northampton, Mass.: Contact Editions. Articles collected from *Contact Quarterly,* 1980–92.

Feldenkrais, Moshe. 1977. *Awareness through movement: Health exercises for personal growth.* New York: Harper and Row. A description of the Feldenkrais approach to learning and moving efficiently. Includes a series of 12 practical lessons.

Franklin, Eric N. 2002. *Relax your neck, liberate your shoulders: The ultimate exercise program for tension relief.* Hightstown, N.J.: Princeton Book Company. Explanations, images, and exercise to help relieve tension in the neck and shoulders.

———. 2003. *Pelvic power: Mind/body exercises for strength, flexibility, posture, and balance for men and women.* Hightstown, N.J.: Princeton Book Company. Explains the role of the pelvic floor muscles in supporting movement and how to train them.

———. 2006. *Inner focus, outer strength: Using imagery and exercise for strength, health and beauty.* Hightstown, N.J.: Princeton Book Company. An overview of the author's approach to making and keeping the human body fit for movement.

Hackney, Peggy. 1998. *Making connections: Total body integration through Bartenieff fundamentals.* Amsterdam: Gordon and Breach. A thorough explanation of a pioneering movement analysis and training system, explained by one of Ms. Bartenieff's students, who is also a co-developer of Integrated Movement Studies.

Hartley, Linda. 1995. *Wisdom of the body moving: An introduction to body-mind centering.* Berkeley, Calif.: North Atlantic. One practitioner's perspective on an approach to movement pioneered by Bonnie Bainbridge Cohen and collaborators.

Jacobson, Edmund. 1938. *Progressive relaxation: An investigation of muscular states and their significance in psychology and medical practice.* 2nd ed. Chicago: University of Chicago Press. The grandfather of modern relaxation techniques explains the background and benefits of using relaxation as a tool for medical treatment and the enhancement of everyday living.

Leivadi, S., M. Hernandez-Reif, T. Field, M. O'Rourke, S. D'Arienzo, D. Lewis, N. del Pino, S. Schanberg, and C. Kuhn. 1999. Massage therapy and relaxation effects on university dance students. *Journal of Dance Medicine & Science* 3 (3): 108–12. A study that analyzes the effects of twice weekly 30-minute massage sessions on dancers.

Pargman, David. 2006. *Managing performance stress: Models and methods.* New York: Routledge. Discusses the elements of stress and how to manage it in performance situations.

Sweigard, Lulu. 1974. *Human movement potential: Its ideokinetic facilitation.* New York: University Press of America. Sweigard was a student of Mabel Todd. This work might be considered an extension of the work described in Todd's book, *The thinking body.*

Todd, Mabel E. 1980. *The thinking body.* Pennington, N.J.: Princeton Book Company. First published in 1929 as *The balancing of forces in the human being.* Combines the author's perspectives on anatomy, physiology, biomechanics, and psychology to create a practical understanding of how the human body moves. Reprint of 1937 revision.

Conditioning, Fitness, Training Systems

Alpers, Amy T., and Rachel T. Segel. 2002. *The everything Pilates book.* Avon, Mass.: Adams Media. Explains the Pilates approach to fitness training and gives in-depth descriptions of a dozen pivotal exercises. Authors are former dancers who run a highly regarded Pilates teacher training center in Boulder, Colorado.

Berardi, Gigi. 1991. *Finding balance: Fitness and training for a lifetime in dance.* Princeton, N.J.: Princeton Book Company. Offers a comprehensive perspective on training for a career in dance, including commentary by well-known professional dancers who have had long careers.

———. 2005. *Finding balance: Fitness and training for a lifetime in dance.* 2nd ed. New York: Routledge. Update and expansion of the 1991 edition with new commentaries.

Bompa, Tudor O. 1999. *Periodization training for sports*. 4th ed. Champaign, Ill.: Human Kinetics. Addresses the topic of training in cycles (pushing hard and backing off) to avoid overtraining, staleness, and injuries.

Calais-Germain, Blandine, and Andree Lamotte. 2008. *Anatomy of movement: Exercises*. Seattle: Eastland Press. Biomechanically wise exercises that follow naturally from explanations offered in Calais-Germain's 2007 book, *Anatomy of Movement*.

Franklin, Eric N. 2004. *Conditioning for dance: Training for peak performance in all dance forms*. Champaign, Ill.: Human Kinetics. Describes an imagery-based approach to dance conditioning, including the use of small exercise balls and elastic bands. The final sections are organized around particular challenges that dancers face.

Isaacs, Benno, and Jay Kobler. 1978. *What it takes to feel good: The Nickolaus technique*. New York: Viking. A combination of Pilates, yoga, and dance exercises integrated into a whole-body exercise program that does make you feel good. One of my favorites, but it is out of print, so you will have to look for it in your local library or a used bookstore.

Isacowitz, Rael. 2006. *Pilates*. Champaign, Ill.: Human Kinetics. A guide to Pilates exercise on the mat and all apparatus by the founder of Body Arts & Science International, a highly regarded Pilates teacher training program. The exercise descriptions and photographs are clear, well organized, and especially instructive.

Koutedakis, Y., L. Myszkewycz, D. Soulas, V. Papapostolou, I. Sullivan, and N. C. C. Sharp. 1999. The effects of rest and subsequent training on selected physiological parameters in professional female classical dancers. *International Journal of Sports Medicine* 20: 379–83. Seventeen ballerinas from the Birmingham Royal Ballet were tested before and after a six-week summer holiday. They improved on several measures of fitness, suggesting that some dancers may be overtraining.

Koutedakis, Yiannis, and N. C. Craig Sharp, eds. 1999. *The fit and healthy dancer*. New York: Wiley. A comprehensive look at dancers' needs with an emphasis on exercise physiology by dance science researchers, one of whom is a former dancer and teacher.

Markgraf, Amy. 1999. *Periodization as a conditioning model for a collegiate modern dance company*. Master's thesis, Brigham Young University, Provo, Utah. Explains the essential features of periodization and how using it might be helpful to dancers. Includes a full-year outline showing how periodization can be used to organize training and rehearsal activities for a modern dance company.

Mattingly, Kate. 2002. A trend toward self-reliance. *Dance Magazine*, November, 38–40. Explains how dancers today have to take responsibility for their own training to prepare for the diversity of demands their bodies are likely to face.

Nagrin, Daniel. 1988. *How to dance forever: Surviving against the odds.* New York: Quill. A personal perspective on what dancers can do to stay healthy, written by a dancer who began a solo career at an age when most dancers retire.

Pilates, Joseph H. 1934, 1998. *Your health: A corrective system of exercising that revolutionizes the entire field of physical education.* Incline Village, Nev.: Presentation Dynamics. A concise text explaining the fundamentals of the training approach that has become the Pilates Method.

Pilates, Joseph H., and William J. Miller. 1945, 2003. *Return to life through Contrology.* Miami: Pilates Method Alliance. Begins with a description of the Pilates approach to exercise. The final two-thirds of the text describes the exercises with photographic demonstrations.

Siler, Brooke. 2000. *The Pilates body.* New York: Broadway Books. Explains the Pilates approach from a contemporary perspective. Includes descriptions and photos of three levels of Pilates mat exercises, as well as easy-to-follow photographic maps of each exercise program.

Sleamaker, Rob. 1989. *Serious training for serious athletes.* Champaign, Ill.: Leisure Press. Designed primarily for endurance athletes, this text describes the advantages of systematic planning and record keeping. Includes an explanation of how to use periodization (training in cycles) to get the most from every workout and avoid burnout.

Watkins, Andrea, and Priscilla M. Clarkson. 1990. *Dancing longer, dancing stronger.* Princeton, N.J.: Princeton Book Company. Describes an exercise program designed to complement dancers' work in technique classes. Essential concepts in anatomy, kinesiology, and physiology are introduced with the exercises.

Injuries, Prevention, Health Care

Arnheim, Daniel D. 1988. *Dance injuries: Their prevention and care.* 2nd ed. Pennington, N.J.: Princeton Book Company. An early classic that describes specific injuries common in dance.

Dishman, Rod K., ed. 1988. *Exercise adherence: Its impact on public health.* Champaign, Ill.: Human Kinetics. New exercise programs are most useful if you continue to do them. This text reviews the research on what it takes to continue an exercise program.

———. 1994. *Advances in exercise adherence.* Champaign, Ill.: Human Kinetics. Update and continuation of the evolving understanding of what it takes to continue an exercise program.

Featherstone, Donald F., and Rona Allen. 1970. *Dancing without danger.* Cranbury, N.J.: A. S. Barnes. An early work written for ballet dancers and teachers to help them understand orthopaedic injuries and how to reduce the risk of sustaining one.

Hagins, Marshall, ed. 2002. *Dance medicine resource guide.* 2nd ed. Andover, N.J.: J. Michael Ryan. A directory of medical practitioners and facilities that specialize in treating dancers, organized by geographic areas throughout the world.

Howse, Justin, and Shirley Hancock. 1988. *Dance technique and injury prevention.*

New York: Routledge. A comprehensive text that begins with anatomy and progresses through technical faults, imbalances, injuries, and treatment. Also includes preventive exercises.

Negus, Vicki, Diana Hopper, and N. Kathryn Briffa. 2005. Associations between turnout and lower extremity injuries in classical ballet dancers. *Journal of Orthopaedic & Sports Physical Therapy* 35 (5): 307–18. Study assessing turnout in Australian professional ballet dancers that suggests the ability to control turnout may be more important than absolute range of motion for avoiding overuse injuries in dance.

Peterson, Lars, and Per Renstrom. 1986. *Sports injuries: Their prevention and treatment.* Chicago: Yearbook Medical. Not specific to dancers, but the clear, colorful drawings of injuries bring the structures and possible damage to life. Ouch!

Pollock, Michael L. 1988. Prescribing exercise for fitness and adherence. In Rod K. Dishman, ed., *Exercise adherence: Its impact on public health,* 259–77. Champaign, Ill.: Human Kinetics. Analysis of a collection of studies on exercise adherence by his local research team. Concludes that working too long (duration) and too hard (intensity) increases the risk of quitting an exercise program.

Ryan, Allan J., and Robert E. Stephens. 1987. *Dance medicine: A comprehensive guide.* Chicago: Pluribus. A collection of chapters written by a variety of dance medicine specialists. Addresses injury epidemiology (origin and pattern) and etiology (causes), training, nutrition, and ailments to each major part of the dancers' body. Considered a classic by dance medicine specialists.

Shantz, Mary P. 1992. *Back care basics.* Berkeley, Calif.: Rodmell. Begins by describing the anatomy of the back and common sources of back pain, and then describes a yoga-based approach to resolving and avoiding back pain.

Solomon, Ruth, John Solomon, and Sandra C. Minton. 2005. *Preventing dance injuries.* Champaign, Ill.: Human Kinetics. A collection of articles by leaders in the field.

Vincent, Larry M. 1988. *The dancer's book of health.* Hightstown, N.J.: Princeton Book Company. An early classic that describes injuries common among dancers and what can be done about them.

Wright, Stuart. 1985. *Dancer's guide to injuries of the lower extremity: Diagnosis, treatment, care.* New York: Cornwall. A practical text that can help dancers determine what they can do for themselves when injured and when to see a health care provider.

New Resources for Dancers

Horosko, Marian, and Judith F. Kupersmith, M.D. 2009. *The dancer's survival manual: Everything you need to know from the first class to career change.* 2nd ed. Gainesville: University Press of Florida. A no-nonsense approach to topics such as choosing a dance school, auditioning, resumes and photographs, makeup, rivalries, and working after leaving the stage.

Hamilton, Linda H., and New York City Ballet, 2008. *The dancer's way: The New York City Ballet guide to mind, body, and nutrition.* New York: St. Martin's Press. A guide to dancer wellness from the perspective of the New York City Ballet.

Video Recordings and Web Sites

An abundance of exercise videotapes and DVDs addressing many of the challenges that dancers face have been produced over the past 10 years. Some are designed for following along, while others are more instruction oriented. Many Web sites provide access to videos, equipment, and training programs relevant to dance conditioning. The recordings and Web site included here are a sample of what is available. The Web sites were last accessed in August 2008.

Dowd, Irene, and Peggy Baker. 2002. *Orbits, spirals, volutes.* Series of three VHS recordings produced by Canada's National Ballet School. <*www.theshoeroom. ca*>. All three choreographies address special challenges dancers face. Orbits contains "Warming up the hip: Turn-out dance."

Isacowitz, Rael. 2006. *Rael Pilates: System 7, 17, 27.* Series of three DVDs by Body Arts and Science International. <*www.basipilates.com/store*>. Pilates mat exercises in three progressive programs.

Krasnow, Donna. 1998. *CI training: Conditioning with imagery.* Series of three VHS/DVDs. <*www.citraining.com*>. Dance professor Donna Krasnow teaches conditioning for dancers at three levels. Includes percussion accompaniment.

Larkham, Elizabeth. 1996. *Balanced body Pilates mat program.* VHS/DVD or NTSC. <*www.pilates.com/BBAPP/V/videos/exercise-video.html*>. Explains and demonstrates correct execution of evolved Pilates mat repertoire in some detail.

New York City Ballet. 2002, 2003. *New York City Ballet workout.* VHS or DVD, Palm Pictures. <*www.nycballet.com/teachers/workout.html*>. Features NYCB dancers and includes personal insights into the dancers' daily lives.

Pilates Pro (online newsletter). <*www.pilates-pro.com*>. Resource for Pilates teachers.

Pilates Style (online newsletter). <*www.pilatesstyle.com/html/newsletter.htm*>. Designed for Pilates enthusiasts.

Rommett, Zena. 1991, 1997, 1999, 2001, 2005. *Zena Rommett Floor-Barre.* Series of five VHS/DVD/PAL recordings, Zena Rommett Dance Foundation. <www. floor-barre.org>. Includes titles designed for professional dancers, young dancers, and athletes.

Solomon, Ruth. 1988. *Anatomy as a master image in training dancers.* VHS/DVD. <http://arts.ucsc.edu/faculty/Solomon/video.html>. A one-hour dance warm-up designed and taught by one of the pioneers of dance medicine and science.

Spector-Flock, Noa. 2001. *Get stronger by stretching.* Hightstown, N.J.: Princeton Book Company. <www.dancehorizons.com>. Series of three videos: center—50 minutes; lower body—63 minutes; upper body—31 minutes. Uses a 6' (2 m) length of elastic band (e.g., Thera-Band®) to resist dancelike movements.

Stott Pilates. 1998–2007. Professional DVD series, Merrithew Entertainment, Toronto. <www.stottpilates.com/store>. The extensive Stott library of exercise videos is clear, easy to follow, and a satisfying balance between instruction and practice. The "Professional" series is in its third edition. The company also offers an "At home" series with emphasis on special topics such as toning and relaxation.

Yoga Journal. Poses. <www.yogajournal.com/poses>. Includes a photo and simple description of each pose with the option to get details such as its anatomical focus, benefits, and prerequisite poses.

Relaxation Recordings

McManus, Carolyn. *Progressive relaxation and autogenic training.* Available through <www.Amazon.com>.

Mind Tools. CDs and MP3s. Available through <www.mindtools.com/stress/RelaxationTechniques/RelaxationTapes.htm>.

Minnick, Heidi. *Guided relaxation: For the body and mind.* Available through <www.Amazon.com>.

Nutrition

My Pyramid <www.mypyramid.gov>

Dance Medicine and Science Resources

Dance UK, Healthy Dancer Programme at <www.danceuk.org/metadot/index.pl>. A model advocacy program for dancers.

Harkness Center for Dance Injuries at <www.med.nyu.edu/hjd/harkness>. Includes a section for students that explains the field and the type of career opportunities it provides.

International Association for Dance Medicine and Science (IADMS) at <www.iadms.org>.

Nureyev Foundation at <www.nureyev.org>. Includes medical information.

Performing Arts Medicine Association at <www.artsmed.org>. Hosts an annual conference and sponsors a journal that addresses medical issues faced by musicians and dancers.

Fitness Teacher Training and Certifying Agencies

Aerobic Fitness Association of America at <www.afaa.com>.

American College of Sports Medicine at <www.acsm.org>.

American Council on Exercise at <www.acefitness.org>.

Associates in Orthopaedics and Sports Medicine at <www.aosmclinic.com>.
National Strength and Conditioning Association at <www.nsca-lift.org>.

Pilates and Gyrotonic® Teacher Training Programs

Body Arts and Science International at <www.basipilates.com>.
Gyrotonic Expansion System: Teacher Training at <www.gyrotonic.com>.
Kane School of Core Integration at *<www.kaneschool.com>*.
Physical Mind Institute at <www.themethodpilates.com>.
Pilates Center of Boulder at <http://thepilatescenter.com>.
Pilates Method Alliance at <www.pilatesmethodalliance.org>.
Polestar Pilates at <www.polestarpilates.com>.
Stott Pilates at <www.stottpilates.com>.

Somatic Training Programs

Body-Mind Centering, Bartenieff Fundamentals, Alexander Technique at <www.
    movingoncenter.org>.
Feldenkrais Method at <www.feldenkrais.com>.
Ideokinesis at <www.ideokinesis.com>.
Integrated Movement Studies at <www.dance.utah.edu/degrees/ims.html>.
Laban Movement Studies at <http://ny.com/dance/laban.html>.

Equipment

Balanced Body at <www.pilates.com/BBAPP/V/home.html>.
Fitness Wholesale at <www.fwonline.com>.
Functional Footprints at <www.functionalfootprints.com>.
Gratz Pilates at <www.pilates-gratz.com>.
Peak Pilates at <www.peakpilates.com>.
Rolling Dance Chair Project at <http://rdc.arts.usf.edu/default.htm>.
Stott Pilates at <www.stottpilates.com>.

Index

Tom Welsh is on the dance faculty at Florida State University in Tallahassee, where he teaches dance conditioning, dance kinesiology, science of dance training, and Pilates for dancers. He conducts research into healthy approaches to training dancers. He served ten years as chair of the research committee for the International Association for Dance Medicine and Science, and he is a member of the editorial board for the *Journal of Dance Medicine & Science.*

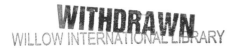